The eNd of 1

THE EXTRAORDINARY BENEFITS OF A
LACTOSE-FREE DIET

CHRIS REESE

Chris Reese/The eNd of 1
Printed in the United States of America

The eNd of 1/ Chris Reese -- 1st ed.

ISBN 9781730793219 Print Edition

CONTENTS

Mom, thank you from the bottom of my heart for believing in me...oh yeah..and for giving me these two holes in my neck.

INTRODUCTION

Welcome to Lactose-Free Living!

Okay – maybe I'm jumping the gun. But I hope that since you've picked up this book, you're interested in learning how and why a lactose-free diet will benefit you.

As I'll explain in these pages, I fell into lactose-free living accidentally. But once I experienced the benefits – and once I began looking into *why* I felt so much better on a lactose-free diet – there was no looking back.

In this book, you'll learn about my lactose-free journey, as well as the journeys of others who chose this path. You'll learn how I formulated a theory about lactose's effect on the immune system. You'll learn why I believe that a properly functioning immune system is the key to *all* health – whether to help our bodies fight something as simple as the common cold or as complex as Parkinson's disease.

Please understand that I am not a doctor or a scientist. I have no scientific evidence of the benefits to the immune system of eating a lactose-free diet. But I do have a theory – and I think it's a good one – about why lactose (which the majority of the human population is unable to break down into simple sugars) clogs the immune system and prevents it from functioning at its best.

To the best of my knowledge, no one in the scientific or medical community has studied this theory. It's certainly not proven – but it's not disproven, either.

Do People Need Lactose?

In my opinion, not only do we *not* need lactose, but lactose is tremendously detrimental to human health.

Why? In these pages you'll learn that:

- Lactose is a disaccharide.
- The enzyme lactase enables the small intestines of young mammals to break down lactose into the simple sugars glucose and galactose.
- Production of lactase stops at weaning for most humans and for essentially every other mammal on the planet.
- Some humans have developed the ability to produce lactase post-weaning. This is called lactase persistence.
- Lactase persistence varies greatly from person to person. It depends on genetics, ethnicity, and age.
- Without lactase, our bodies cannot break down lactose.
- In my opinion, intact lactose has a profoundly detrimental effect on immune system functions.
- The immune system is the key to all health.
- Lactose-free living enables the lymphatic system (a primary part of the immune system) to:
  - Use its "trash collectors" to **clear out cellular waste**
  - Get to work **repairing damaged body parts**
  - Send in its strongest "soldiers" to **fight disease**

A Word About Ethnicity and Age

I'm of Northern European descent – mostly Norwegian, with a little German thrown in. As you read this book, you'll learn about my story and the stories of a variety of other people who have chosen a lactose-free diet.

In most cases, I'll tell you the person's ethnicity and age. This is important because the ability to produce the enzyme lactase varies greatly based on ethnicity and age.

Humans, like all mammals, drink mother's milk as first food. That milk – whether from a cow or a human female – contains lactose. In order for the infant's body to use the lactose, it must be broken down by lactase into glucose and galactose.

Among many ethnic groups, most members of the group stop producing lactase as toddlers (the general age of weaning). In other groups, particularly among Northern Europeans, lactase persistence (the body's ability to continue producing lactase) continues into childhood – and, for some people, into adulthood. *But I believe that lactase production ceases for **every individual** at some point – and this is when a person's health issues are most likely to arise.*

There is no set formula for lactase persistence, but there are general trends among ethnic groups. Because of this, ethnicity and age are vital to the discussion of lactose-free living.

Tell Me More…

Interested in learning more? Keep reading – and thanks for joining me on this journey!

Chris

CHAPTER 1

ACCIDENTALLY LACTOSE-FREE

How Did This Happen?

It was December of 2016. My wife, Shelly, and I had looked forward for months to this time. We were headed out on a nine-day cruise with my son and daughter, Shelly's son, and several other family members and friends.

Shelly and I, both in our forties, had prepared for the trip the way many our age would – by trying to get in shape. Every day, we worked out in our home gym. We downed protein shakes like they were water. Our goal was to be buff and fit – at least, as buff and fit as two busy, middle-aged parents can be – when we departed for our seagoing adventure.

The cruise proved to be everything we'd hoped for and more – fun times with family and friends, relaxation, sightseeing. The food was great. Every morning, my eleven-year-old son, also named Chris, would head to the large, sumptuous buffet on the lido deck and return to our cabin with a plate of fresh fruit. We'd all enjoy the fruit, along with the view, on our cabin's balcony. Among many recollections, this stands out as a happy pattern that persisted for the entire trip.

Back home in Arizona, we were filled with memories – not to mention a bit of regret about having to return to the "real world."

I resumed my job at a local casino, dealing blackjack. Casinos are pretty much the only places left in the country where people can smoke indoors. I don't smoke, but every day, about an hour after getting to work, my nose would begin to run and I would start to feel congested, due to the cigarette smoke. I was accustomed to keeping plenty of tissues nearby, because I knew that no matter how many allergy pills I took, my congested nose would dribble onto the table if I didn't stay on top of blowing it. This was normal for me and I thought nothing of it.

Except it didn't happen. That first night back at work – and every night since – my nose was clear and dry.

This is so weird, I thought. Was it simply the benefits of vacation – the lack of stress, the family time? Could something that simple cure congestion?

But I was back in my routine now. Logically, my congestion should have returned when we got home from the cruise.

And then I remembered something: a conversation I'd had some months prior with a friend who was staying with us while passing through town. He'd mentioned that he used to have congestion and when he gave up dairy, the problem disappeared.

I realized that when we left on the cruise, we'd stopped drinking our dairy-based protein shakes – and we hadn't gotten back to them when we returned home. On the cruise, we'd enjoyed those fresh fruit plates and a variety of other delicious foods. But I couldn't remember eating much, if any, dairy.

Thinking further about it, I realized I'd heard my friend's same words before. I couldn't remember where or who said them to me, but I did recall hearing stories about people who cleared up their congestion by eating a dairy-free diet.

I hadn't made a conscious choice to do that, but maybe it had happened anyway.

The Dairy-Free Game

At home, I told Shelly what I'd heard, and her interest was piqued, too. She didn't suffer the congestion issues that I did, but she's an overall fit person who is always looking for ways to improve her health.

We began looking at the products in our kitchen cabinets and refrigerator, to see what contained milk. This was easier than you'd think. I didn't know it then, but the Food Allergen Labeling and Consumer Protection Act (FALCPA), which went into effect in 2006, means that all food labels in the United States must state if the product contains – among other allergens – milk. We found numerous products with those words on their labels: "CONTAINS MILK."

We tossed out every one of them.

It kind of became a game for us. We showed each other product after product.

"Look at this one!"

"Can you believe there's milk in these crackers?"

"Can you believe there *isn't* milk in these cookies?"

At the time, we knew nothing about lactose. We didn't even know what lactose was, really. We were just looking for products that contain milk.

Four Weeks Later

By the four-week mark from the time we embarked on the cruise, I'd started to feel like something extraordinary was happening. My congestion was completely gone – with not a single allergy pill ingested. I was breathing like I'd never been able to breathe in my life. I was noticing other benefits, too – I had more energy, felt more focused, and had dropped a few pounds.

With one exception, I'd changed nothing about my diet or routine. The exception was this: in the weeks we'd been home, I hadn't touched any dairy. And although I wasn't completely sure I'd had no dairy on the cruise, I knew that if I'd had any, it was only a trace amount.

Could there be a connection?

Are We Crazy?

Shelly was feeling great, too – better than she had in years. The upper respiratory infections that had plagued her for years disappeared. She lost weight. She even had a bizarre thing happen: in the past when she got hiccups, they were almost violent in force. Now, out of nowhere, she began hiccupping six or seven times, relatively calmly, like a regular person. We laughed about it, but we had to wonder – is there a connection?

Although we wanted to tell everyone, we kept it to ourselves. We were sure that if we told people that we thought there was a connection between ingesting dairy and our overall health, they'd tell us we were crazy.

Our Decision

A month after we'd begun our sea voyage, Shelly and I knew we were ready to embark on a new, very different type of adventure.

If this is what dairy does to you, we decided, there is no way we're going to touch that stuff ever again.

Chris's Lactose-Free Takeaways

Becoming "accidentally dairy-free," I learned that:

- *Taking dairy out of my diet rapidly eliminated health issues* that had annoyed me, but I'd thought of as relatively normal.

- While there's milk in much packaged food, *it's easy to determine if a product contains milk.*
- *It wasn't just me!* Others had also experienced the benefits of removing dairy from their diets.

CHAPTER 2

WHO I AM – AND HOW I'VE CHANGED

My Idyllic Childhood

The seventh of nine kids in a Catholic family, I was born and raised in Greenbush, Minnesota. My heritage is mostly Norwegian, with a little German on my dad's side. (I should mention that all of my siblings are biological siblings, so they have the same heritage as me. This is important to note, because I'll share stories about some of my siblings in later chapters of this book.)

No one could ask for a better upbringing than my brothers, sisters, and I had. Greenbush is a small town (population: 800), right in the middle of dairy country. My parents were married for sixty-one years, until my dad passed away not long ago. We had meat and potatoes – with milk and butter, of course – at every meal. In the wintertime, my mom loved making us kids hot chocolate, using powdered milk.

During the school year, I spent countless afternoons and weekends at friends' dairy farms, helping out. For them it was chores, but I was a "town kid" and working on a farm was fun for me. Looking at those dairy families now, many of the kids I grew up with aren't in the best shape these days. They're in wheelchairs, or they have drain plugs behind the ears, or there's some other kind of health issue. Reflecting now on how much dairy they've been ingesting since a young age makes me wonder what their bodies have gone through, over the years.

My dad owned a construction company and wherever he was building a road in the summertime, he'd get a lake cabin and a golf membership at the nearest resort or club. He'd dump us kids off at about seven in the morning and pick us up at the end of his workday. We got to fish and swim, and we learned how to play a golf a little better than many people do.

Moving Away – and Into Adulthood

Maybe because of those early opportunities, I became rather adept at the game of golf. I went to Mesa Community College in Arizona on a golf scholarship. After college I worked as a golf professional, and I was also a coach for the Central Arizona College golf program.

After many years coaching and teaching golf, I was ready for a change. When the opportunity to work as a blackjack dealer in a casino came along, I jumped at it. I love the casino life. My co-workers are fantastic people, the job pays well, and it's a rewarding way to spend my days and nights.

I've been married three times and I have two kids: Mikkella, a daughter who's now twenty-three with my first wife, and Chris, an eleven-year-old son with my second wife. Shelly, my wife now, also has a twenty-two year-old son – my stepson, Dallas. Additionally, we have a cat and a dog.

Middle Age Hits Home

I'm forty-eight now, and about a decade ago is when I started to see the effects of middle age on my body. At thirty-eight, I began taking erectile dysfunction medication – something no man wants to admit to, but it's key to this story and worth mentioning. (*How* is it key? Keep reading to find out!)

Around that same time, other stuff happened, too. My hair started to thin and fall out. My eyesight got worse. These were little things – stuff that I attributed to approaching forty.

At the same time, I was becoming concerned about the "big things" – namely, heart disease. To put it mildly, heart disease runs rampant in my family. Everybody has arterial clogging; that's where our genetic dams are weak.

My father's heart health was not great. And two of my uncles on my mom's side, as well as my grandfather, all died of heart attacks when they were in their early fifties.

In the midst of these years, my oldest brother, Chinny, died of a his second heart attack, at age fifty-six. (He had his first heart attack in his late forties.) Two other older brothers, Phillip and Luke, also had a heart attacks, at ages forty-seven and fifty-one, respectively. They survived, but the issue was clearly present for them.

So now I was seeing my older brothers have heart attacks. It wasn't just my grandfather, my dad, my uncles. I thought about this a lot, and it made me want to do whatever I could to ensure I didn't follow in their footsteps.

In late 2016, when we went on that cruise I mentioned, I was forty-six. I was well aware – aren't we all? – that here comes fifty, with all its issues: big ones like heart disease, not to mention the small ones that everyone faces, in one form or another.

They tell you stuff will happen to you – and it's no surprise that for most people, it does.

Why? They say it's "just aging" -- but I believe it's all due to lactose.

Three Months of Being Lactose-Free:
Results from Head to Toe

Three months after I stopped eating dairy completely, I took an inventory of what had changed in me:

- Oily forehead – gone
- Dandruff – gone
- Thinning hair filled out
- Snoring – gone
- Gum inflammation – gone
- Mental clarity increased
- Energy increased
- Emotions felt more intensely
- Singing voice improved *(crazy, right?)*
- Sweating after eating – gone
- Congestion – gone
- Coughing – gone
- Eczema – gone
- Warts – gone
- Joint pain – gone
- Erectile dysfunction – gone
- Easier bowel movements
- Weight loss (twenty-five pounds without trying)
- Ceased taking hypertension and erectile dysfunction medicine

Some of the changes – like the absence of congestion and being able to stop taking my erectile dysfunction medication – were momentous for me, as they represented huge improvements to my quality of life. Others – like warts and eczema disappearing with no treatment involved, or a much-improved singing voice – were noticeable and simply made me happy.

I remember visiting my dentist for my biannual checkup, about six months after I went dairy-free. He said, "What are you doing that's different?" Before responding, I asked him why he was asking me this question. He replied, "Every time I've seen you – for years – your gums have been inflamed. Today, there's zero inflammation."

With all the other improvements I'd seen, I wasn't surprised that my gum health had improved as well. In fact, at that point, nothing was surprising me anymore.

I knew dairy was the culprit, and I told the dentist as much. I'm not sure he believed me, but every time I've seen him since, I've had no gum inflammation whatsoever. In fact, I had a dental appointment recently and a new hygienist mentioned how healthy my gums are. I told the hygienist (and reminded the dentist, when he arrived in the room) what had happened to me a year before, in the very chair where I was now sitting. They both said the whole thing is pretty cool!

The mental clarity, however, is the issue that stands out the most for me. I don't know how to describe it, except to say that my mind is more astute, alert, and focused than it's ever been in my life. My memory is sharp. Intelligible thoughts and ideas come quickly to me, and I can articulate them when speaking to others – a huge thing for someone like me, who previously had never been completely comfortable expressing himself in spoken word. It feels like a fog – one I never realized was there – has been lifted.

I don't think it's a coincidence that every person I've talked to who also went 100% dairy-free has mentioned (among other health improvements) the same thing: mental clarity.

Feeling Like a Kid Again

These days, I feel like I can do anything. I remember one day, a few months into my dairy-free diet, I told my stepson, Dallas, "It's been twenty-five years since I dunked a basketball – since I even tried. But I bet I can dunk now."

We went to the gym, and I'll be damned. Dallas threw me an Alley Oop and I slammed her down. I was forty-six years old at the time. How many ex-NBA players of that age can still dunk a ball? And I did it after twenty-five years. I wasn't even working out or trying to get back into shape. It was just me thinking, "Man, I feel like I can jump"— and I could.

That dunk was easy; it was nothing. It was like I was a kid again. *Everything* is like I'm a kid again.

I feel like I'm getting younger by the day.

Lactose-Free Stories: *Young Chris*

My son's name is Chris. He's not a junior, and he'd probably hate that I'm calling him "Young Chris" in this book, but for the sake of clarity, let's call him that.

One thing I love about kids his age – he's eleven – is that they're old enough to think critically but young enough to at least consider what their parents have to say. When I told Young Chris that I was no longer eating dairy – and explained why – he said it made a lot of sense and he wanted to try it, too.

At my house this is easy, because Shelly and I keep no dairy in our kitchen. But Young Chris is only with me part of the time, so I have to rely on my ex-wife – and Young Chris's own judgment – to manage his diet when he's not with me. My ex-wife buys almond milk for Young Chris, and he avoids dairy whenever he can – he doesn't drink milk at school, for instance. But he's a kid – it's hard to be 100% dairy-free when you're a kid going to birthday parties where there's cake with ice cream.

Nonetheless, he gives it his best, and even without being completely dairy-free, there have been benefits. He sleeps soundly all night now. He attributes this to his mouth being more comfortable. His tongue used to get horribly cracked, especially at night, and the pain would keep him up. The cracked tongue has disappeared on a lactose-free diet.

Previously, on our drive to school, Young Chris would clear his throat repeatedly, sounding like he had a frog stuck in there. This trait has vanished. His sclera – the white part of the eye – is snow-white and clear. He's getting A's and B's in school. He was a good student before, but his learning is more focused now. He plays football with kids two years older than him, and he got "Most Improved Player" on the team last year.

Young Chris doesn't say, "Oh, I'm better now at sports and schoolwork." He doesn't see that. But I do.

Lactose-Free Stories: *Ponce de Leon*

I love the story of Ponce de Leon discovering the Fountain of Youth. I realize a lot of it is probably myth – but myth comes from somewhere, right? Perhaps there *is* a grain of truth to it.

The legend is that when Ponce de Leon discovered Florida, he thought he'd found the Fountain of Youth. Why did he think that? Because the older natives – people in their sixties and seventies – looked like they were thirty years old.

He asked himself, "How can they be this old and still so vigorous? What's in the water here?"

But it wasn't about the water at all. It was about their diet. Native Americans, before white settlers came here, did not have dairy. They subsisted on hunting, fishing, gathering, and a little bit of crop farming. Milking an animal was unheard-of. Cattle are not indigenous to North America – and nobody was going around milking indigenous species like buffalo, moose, and bighorn sheep.

Native people didn't have anything in their diets that compromised their health and made them look and act old by the time they were forty – you know, the way many people on a typical western diet look today.

No wonder our buddy Ponce thought he'd discovered the Fountain of Youth! He discovered the Fountain of Lactose-Free Living.

Chris's Lactose-Free Takeaways

Thinking about my own health history, I realized that:

- **A lactose-free diet gave me amazing physical and mental health results** within a short period of time.
- Even if you're relatively fit, **health issues are likely to catch up with you by middle age**.
- Having a history of **serious illness in one's family** (like heart disease) is **cause for concern**.

CHAPTER 3

WHY IS THIS HAPPENING?

What Does Milk Do to Me?

So what did I think of all these changes to my system? You'd
expect me to be thrilled, right?

And I was – who wouldn't be? – but more than elation, what
I experienced was curiosity. I couldn't for the life of me understand why and how eating a dairy-free diet could have such dramatic effects on my physical health and mental state.

It's notable that, at this point, I wasn't thinking about lactose.
I knew very little about lactose, except that it was found in dairy
products. I knew that some people are lactose intolerant. But I
hadn't made the connection that lactose was the culprit. I just
knew I felt much, much better without dairy in my diet.

I'm a naturally curious person; if you give me a riddle or put
a puzzle in front of me, I'm going to try to solve it. This was no
different.

I asked myself – *if milk was making me so unhealthy, why is
that?*

Am I Lactose Intolerant? What Is Lactose Intolerance?

When I looked up "dairy-free diet," tons of articles about lactose
intolerance came up. I learned that lactose is present in cow's

milk and every other mammal's milk, including human milk. As I'd already known, lactose intolerance people are unable to drink cow's milk. I was surprised to learn that some lactose intolerant individuals cannot drink milk from other animals, either, such as sheep or goats.

My understanding – and my research confirmed this – had always been that lactose intolerant people had gastrointestinal issues if they ate dairy, because their bodies couldn't digest it. I didn't know why or how lactose caused digestive problems in some people, but in any case, it didn't apply to me. I could eat dairy with no gastric issues whatsoever.

So if it wasn't lactose intolerance, what was it?

What is Lactase Persistence?

Diving deeper into the data about lactose intolerance, I learned about a trait that many people have but that I'd never before heard of: *lactase persistence.*

Lactase persistence is the ability to continue breaking down lactose into glucose and galactose after weaning.

What does that mean? Lactose is a disaccharide. That means it's a sugar molecule consisting of two other molecules; these are glucose and galactose. Human bodies – like every other mammal's – are incapable of using lactose in its complete form. In order to be used by the body, lactose needs to be broken down into glucose and galactose.

To do that, the small intestine secretes the enzyme *lactase.* The lactase cleaves to the lactose and breaks it down into glucose and galactose, which are then carried from the small intestine to other areas of the body for use – they provide energy and help with growth. All infant mammals secret lactase and thus have the ability to break down the lactose in their mother's milk.

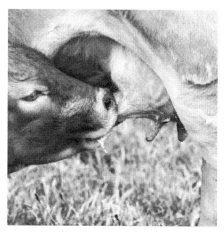

Totally natural: infant mammals (like this calf) receive nourishment from their mother's milk.

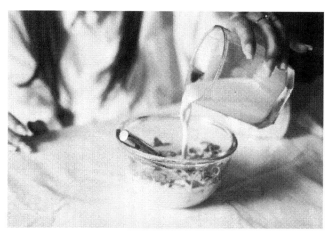

Not-so-natural: pouring milk intended for a calf onto your morning cereal.

Every other mammal on the planet – besides humans – stops producing lactase once it's weaned. This is because there is no lactose in an animal's diet after weaning. So there is no need for the body to keep making lactase.

Humans – some of us, anyway – are different. Many humans continue producing lactase into adulthood. This is an adaptive trait – it happened over thousands of years in certain human populations, particularly those in northern Europe.

Social scientists have theorized that northern Europeans developed lactase persistence because they lived in a cold, dark climate where they were unable to get much Vitamin D from the sun. I can't imagine what they, as a population, went through to get to this state – but over time, people who drank milk from another mammal in these climates evolved to continue producing lactase. Because of this, milk from cows, sheep, and other animals was digestible by this population into adulthood. This pattern has existed for much of the time humans have inhabited the northern areas of Europe.

The map below shows lactase persistence in the indigenous populations of much of the world. (Note that the United States is not shown. But being the "melting pot" that we are, the U.S. does not provide an accurate representation of lactase persistence.)

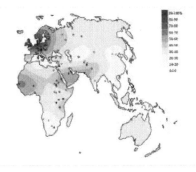

Lactose Intolerance in the Old World

The darkest areas – concentrated around northern Europe – show indigenous populations that are most strongly lactase persistent. Lighter areas show populations that are less lactase persistent.

Notice how light the shading is in most of Africa and Asia? That's because those populations never developed the ability to continue producing lactase into adulthood. (An exception is western Africa, where cattle are prevalent and milk-drinking is more typical.)

As the map moves away from areas that need extra sunlight, less and less people eat dairy. Not coincidentally, less and less people are lactase persistent.

I found this fascinating, but I didn't see how it related to me. Since I'm of northern European descent, if there's anybody that should be able to drink this stuff and not see any ill-effects, it's me.

If Northern Europeans Are Lactase Persistent, Why Do They Get Sick?

As noted above, northern Europeans developed lactase persistence as an evolutionary trait. Physiologically, it enhanced their survival. Milk from an animal was an easy food to acquire. It stored well (inside the animal), it could be converted into other products like butter and cheese – and, as long as one continued to feed and care for the animal, there was a continually replenishing supply. It's no surprise that people in this part of the world evolved to rely on it.

However, I think it's a fallacy to believe that because you're of northern European descent, you can have as much dairy as you like and still live a long, healthy life. Just because your ancestors were Vikings doesn't mean your small intestine will continue to secret lactase for the rest of your life.

How do I know this? I don't, for sure – but I do know that health issues seem to catch up with just about everyone – *even those of northern European descent* – by the time people are forty or fifty years old.

Think about the middle aged people you know. How many of them have something they're dealing with, health-wise? I'll bet it's a good number.

Why? Because for thousands of years, a life expectancy of forty or fifty was the norm for northern Europeans. Did they become seriously ill at that point? A lot of them did – and throughout most of history, there was no modern medicine keeping people alive after serious illness invaded their bodies.

Look up the onset age for serious diseases. For children up to age ten, you might see a little sliver. For older kids and teens, perhaps a bigger sliver – and for people in their twenties and thirties, again a bit bigger sliver.

And then – bam, everything happens when you get to forty and beyond. For example, 25% of new cancer cases are diagnosed in people aged sixty-five to seventy-four.

Who *doesn't* it happen to? People who don't eat dairy.

Need proof? A recent study shows that vegan women had 34% lower rates of female-specific cancers such as breast, cervical, and ovarian cancer than their non-vegan counterparts. And Asian/Pacific Islander women (who in general eat little or no dairy) have the lowest cancer mortality rate among all adults in the United States, when comparing groups based on ethnicity and gender.

So what's happening here? What I believe is that we've created a fiction that "falling apart" at middle age is just part of the process.

Have you seen this one on social media?

Welcome to your 40s. If you do not already have a mysterious ailment, one will be assigned to you shortly.

We laugh at things like this on social media. But are they true?

We all might nod our heads, thinking, "Yep, that's just the way it is." But in my view, that's a myth – certainly for the bulk of western society, and probably for the bulk of the world.

Lactose-Free Stories: Aaron Rodgers and Tom Brady

Like many Americans, I like watching football. And like anyone who follows the game, I know there are only thirty-two quarterbacks who are starters on an NFL team, and out of those thirty-two, only about five of them are truly incredible. The best of the best right now? For my money, it's Aaron Rodgers and Tom Brady.

Think about the types of split-second decisions Rodgers and Brady have to make. How do they make it look so effortless? What's going through their minds?

I began to wonder what people like that eat.

I knew that Tom Brady has a book out, trying to sell his fitness plan to people. What does he say we should eat? Well, Brady is not just dairy-free – he's everything-free. GMOs, sugar, white flour, caffeine, even fruit – you name it and Brady likely doesn't eat it.

The key for me, though, is that Brady has been consuming a lactose-free diet for a long time.

Brady claims he'll play football until he's forty-five years old. Some QBs in the league can't make it past thirty; they're too beat up. But Brady seems unstoppable. Could his power and skills be related to his diet? I absolutely believe they are.

In my opinion, Aaron Rodgers's strength and decision-making skills rival Brady's. So what does Rodgers eat? I decided to find out. Sure enough – even playing in "America's Dairyland," Rodgers has been lactose-free for over two years.

Rodgers has said that inflammation can be reduced via proper diet. He maintains that some foods increase inflammation in the body. Post knee-surgery, he says, he began thinking more carefully about what he was eating.

And what did he give up? Well, let's just say Aaron Rodgers couldn't call himself a Cheesehead if the term was based on what he eats.

Lactose-Free Stories: Thomas Edison

I'll admit it; I've had some fun researching the diets of famous people. After Brady and Rodgers, the next person I looked into was Thomas Edison.

Have you ever been to a chiropractor? If you have, I'll bet you've seen this quote hanging in the chiropractor's office:

"The doctor of the future will give no medication, but will interest his patients in the care of the human frame, in diet and in the cause and prevention of disease." – Thomas Edison

A famous quote attributed to Thomas Edison.

Edison believed that nutrition and preventative care, not medicine, were the keys to our health. Because of this, I figured he probably stuck to a flawless diet. His wife, Mina, has been quoted as saying that correct eating was one of his greatest hobbies.

I don't know exactly what he ate, but I did learn one tidbit. Popular lore is that in the last few years of his life, Edison swore by a fad diet: the only liquid he consumed was a pint of milk every three hours. He believed drinking nothing but milk would restore his health.

Not long afterward, Edison died of complications from diabetes.

Chris's Lactose-Free Takeaways
Exploring why I felt better on a dairy-free diet, I discovered:
- **Lactase persistence** – the body's ability to digest and use lactose – **varies throughout the world's population**.
- Even those with lactase persistence **might not have this trait for the entirety of their lives**.
- People who eat **little or no dairy tend to live longer and healthier lives**.

CHAPTER 4

HOW DO OUR BODIES USE LACTOSE?

My Theory

I want to begin this chapter by stating that what I'm saying here (and in the subsequent two chapters – and really, throughout this book) is *my theory*. It's based on my own and others' results on a lactose-free diet, as well as non-scientific research I've done.

My goal in writing this book – and speaking about this topic whenever I get the opportunity – is for these ideas to come to the attention of the scientific community. I'd like nothing more than to see thorough clinical research conducted on this subject.

Could Lactose be Causing Problems Besides Digestion Issues? And If So, How?

Going back to the dairy-free diet information I talked about in Chapter 3, I noticed a common theme: while all of the articles discussed how removing dairy from one's diet provides relief from the gastrointestinal issues caused by lactose intolerance, many of them also mentioned other benefits: *clearer skin, less congestion, increased energy.* These were the types of benefits I'd seen. None of my issues that resolved themselves on a dairy-free diet were digestion-related.

I began to wonder if there could be a connection between lactose ingestion and overall health.

Digging further, I looked into the causes and effects of what had been my most pressing issues: congestion and erectile dysfunction. I also looked into the smaller issues, such as gum inflammation and eczema, which had resolved themselves on my dairy-free diet.

Over and over, I found the same thing mentioned: every one of these issues was related to the immune system. A properly functioning immune system, I learned, is what the body uses to resolve issues and irregularities – from a stuffy nose to inflamed gums to problems for guys in the bedroom.

My Curious Trait: Branchial Cleft Fistulas

While researching the immune system, I came across the medical term for an odd, lifelong feature of my body – two small holes in my neck. I've had them all my life. I learned that such holes are called **branchial cleft fistulas**. The development of this condition is the equivalent of a gill system of a fish – but in humans they're considered a birth defect. They're rare, and many people who have them do not have the holes, so they experience swelling that may have to be surgically drained. Mine never swelled, but – brace yourself for grossness – if I got an upper respiratory or sinus infection, the fistulas would expel mucus that looks like what comes out of a little kid's snotty nose.

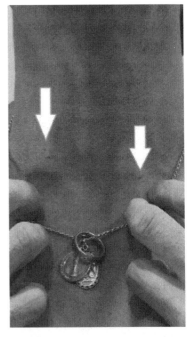

The arrows in this figure are pointing to my branchial cleft fistulas.

I was used to this; I'd had this condition my entire life. To most people it would seem like an oddity, but it was normal for me.

However, when I stopped eating dairy, my brachial cleft fistulas stopped expelling that disgusting mucus. Now, if anything came out at all, it was clear, and was only a drop or two. In the same way that my congestion cleared up on a dairy-free diet, so also did my brachial cleft fistulas "clear up."

Reading further, I learned that branchial cleft fistulas are a direct line to the lymphatic system, which is part of the immune system. The mucus that mine were expelling was simply lymph, which is the fluid produced by the lymphatic system. This fluid – which, when it's healthy, is clear or somewhat whitish – consists of white blood cells. (Note: There is much more about the lymphatic system in Chapter 5.)

But the condition of my lymph had been appalling. It felt unhealthy and it looked even worse. On my dairy-free diet, I was glad to see that stuff out of my system.

The fact that poor-quality lymph was no longer gushing out of me seemed like a good thing. But it made me wonder: where is my new-and improved lymph going instead? And how is it being used?

Was it possible, I wondered, that my lymphatic system was functioning more efficiently on a dairy-free diet than it had when I was routinely ingesting lactose?

About Digesting Lactose

To review what we talked about so far, keep in mind:

- *Lactose is a disaccharide* – a sugar composed of two molecules. These two molecules are glucose and galactose.

- No matter what mammal you are, unless the enzyme lactase in your small intestine breaks lactose in into glucose and galactose, *lactose cannot be used at a cellular level.*
- Many people with ancestry in Europe maintain lactase production into adulthood. This is an evolutionary trait called *lactase persistence.*

I Still Eat Sugar

Are you surprised? You might be even more surprised to learn that I love Skittles. I'll bet I consume one of those two-pound bags of Skittles nearly every week!

Sounds pretty unhealthy, right? But remember that sugar is just sugar. It's a fuel. Whether you eat a banana or a Skittle, your body is going to use it the same way – as energy.

The key is that in order for the body to use it, a sugar must be a *simple sugar* – in other words, a singular molecule of sugar, not a disaccharide like lactose.

Lactose, when it's broken down into glucose and galactose, is used the same way as other simple sugars. Just like any other "ose," glucose and galactose are simple sugars. In their singular molecular form, they're used by the body in the same way as fructose or any other simple sugar.

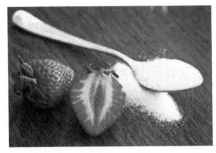

No matter what "ose" it is, sugar is just sugar.

The problem, per se, isn't the "ose" in lactose. The problem isn't that lactose – or even glucose and galactose – are sugar molecules.

The problem is that ***most human bodies cannot break down lactose into a usable, simple form of energy.***

How Big is Your Cheeseburger?

Visualize a cheeseburger on your plate. (It's okay – for this exercise, you can even visualize the cheese.) Now imagine you're starving, so instead of a single, you order a double cheeseburger. It's perfect and you devour every bite.

Let's take it one step further. Suppose you order a double cheeseburger, but your server brings you a quadruple cheeseburger instead. You take one look and realize there's no way you can eat that thing without breaking it into smaller pieces.

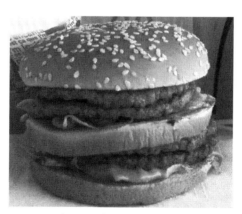

A bit much for most of us...

Now suppose that for some reason, you're unable to break it apart. In this case, you wouldn't even attempt to eat it. No matter how hungry you were, if what was on your plate was a rock-solid quadruple cheeseburger, you wouldn't eat it. You'd just throw it away and eat something else instead.

This is what a body that no longer produces lactase has to do with lactose.

Lactose-Free Stories: *Quentin*

I love telling people about Quentin, because he's like a son to me. Seeing how his health has improved on a lactose-free diet brings me incredible joy.

Quentin is my stepson Dallas's best friend. Quentin and Dallas were kids together just outside Louisville, Kentucky – they lived in southern Indiana. Quentin's heritage is half Asian and half white. He's highly asthmatic; as a kid, he was tied to an inhaler. His asthma meant that his friendship with Dallas revolved around games and stuff you can do inside.

My wife moved to Arizona when Dallas was ten, but in this day and age, you can still have a best friend two thousand miles away. You might not be playing together every day, but you stay in close contact. After high school, Quentin moved to Arizona, and he and Dallas got an apartment together.

One night a few months after I began my dairy-free lifestyle, I got a call about Quentin. He was in the hospital, at Desert Sam. I went to see him right away. He had been diagnosed with pneumonia and was on a ventilator. Shelly and I were looking out for this kid – as I mentioned, he's like a son to us. I *hated* seeing him like that.

I started thinking about how Quentin had said congestion causes him to get this way – and, he told us, it happens often. He was smoking, even though he knew better, and certainly that contributed to his landing in the hospital. Regardless, when he was able to talk, I phoned him.

"I don't know what's going on," I told Quentin. "I took dairy out of my diet and things have changed in me so greatly that I feel compelled to tell you about it. I don't know if you want to try it, but you're the first person I thought of when it comes to this."

He replied, "If this can help my asthma, I'll try it."

After that, I didn't talk to him for about a month. Then I called one day to check on him.

"Man," he said. "I'm using my puffer less and I'm spitting less. All this stuff that used to come up – it's getting better. I think you might be right about this."

At the three month mark of eating a lactose-free diet, Quentin experienced the following:

- No using or even carrying an inhaler
- Spitting little to no phlegm (absolutely huge for an asthmatic individual)
- Better overall breathing, due to lack of phlegm production
- Cessation of taking allergy medication
- Better focus and mental clarity
- Almost complete removal of sluggish feeling in the morning
- Able to play basketball for three hours at a time

Today, Quentin is still 100% lactose-free.

In his own words: "After speaking with Chris, I executed a plan to remove lactose from my diet, solely trusting his word. Some of my results were expected (by Chris), while some were new to the both of us because I am a different person with different issues. I'm very excited that some of my lifelong issues have changed. This is an outstanding basis for an experimental diet. I've had two or three common colds since I started feeling better due to my lactose-free diet. I was able to recover from two of these colds with no prescribed medicine – a tremendous improvement for me. For the third, I had strep throat and needed medication, but I didn't even need to take the full round before I was healed. My body is so much stronger and less prone to becoming overwhelmed when fighting sickness."

I think back to Quentin's frustration with his health for so many years. I have no idea how many years he's added to his life, but I am absolutely certain his dramatic health improvements are tied to his commitment to a lactose-free diet.

Lactose-Free Stories: *Garrick and Jade*

My favorite stories are about people who go 100% lactose free, because I firmly believe that going 100% makes exponentially more difference than giving up some dairy, but not all.

Two such people are Garrick and Jade. They're both in their early twenties. Garrick is three-quarters African-American and one-quarter white. Jade, his girlfriend, is mostly white, with a little bit of Native American heritage. Garrick is my wife Shelly's cousin. He's an aspiring rapper and he's pretty good! Shelly and I go to the Kentucky Derby most years, and it's always a big reunion of family and friends. We've been seeing Jade and Garrick there for years.

The Derby is the first weekend in May, so when we went in 2017, we'd been dairy-free for over four months. Shelly mentioned to me that she'd heard Garrick had been having stomach problems. It sounded like an opportunity to me, so I had a chat with him.

I said, "I heard you've been having some belly issues."

"Man," Garrick replied, shaking his head. "I've been throwing up a few times a week and I have no idea why. It sucks."

At that point I'd put together a presentation of sorts on my discoveries about lactose. I pulled it up on my laptop to show him.

When I finished, Garrick was thoughtful.

"You know," he said. "When I started to get sick, when I started having these issues, is when I came up with the idea that after track practice, I'd come home and have two big bowls of cereal. I've been doing that every day. Now, looking back at all the milk that I started drinking that I wasn't drinking before, I can see that it could have something to do with my stomach."

He gave me a long look. "You've convinced me," he said. "I'll try this."

It's been over a year now, and this is Garrick's health update:

- Less mucus
- Better breathing
- No stomach swelling
- Rare vomiting
- Rare diarrhea
- Better bowel movements
- Less body temperature fluctuations
- Better hair and nail growth
- No acne or oily skin
- Healthy weight loss
- More energy
- Clear, more creative mind

Garrick is so convinced, he's become a walking advertisement for lactose-free living. He had shirts printed with the words: LACTOSE FREE. He posts on social media with the hashtag #lactosefree. He's more committed to this issue right now than he is to his music. He feels the effects of lactose are particularly harmful for African-Americans – which is true; next to Native

Americans, African Americans have the highest rates of lactose intolerance in the United States. Garrick believes (and I agree with him) that the number of African Americans who are undiagnosed lactose intolerant is very, very high.

Jade didn't have pressing health issues, but she starting eating a lactose-free diet when Garrick did, because the reasoning makes sense to her. I saw her a few months ago, and she's lost more than twenty-five pounds. She looks like a supermodel. I'd never say anyone should stop eating dairy purely to lose weight – but it's a nice side benefit, especially for individuals like Jade who had no serious health concerns but just wanted to improve their overall health and wellbeing.

Jade's father is on a kidney transplant list, and she's talked to him about this. He's still a young man. He's part Native American, so it's very likely his body no longer produces lactase – if it ever did.

So far, Jade's father isn't interested in going lactose-free. We're hopeful, though.

Chris's Lactose-Free Takeaways

As I learned how the body uses lactose, I concluded that:

- There is a **connection between lactose ingestion and overall immune health.**
- A curious physical trait of mine could be a clue that **links my lactose-free diet to my lymphatic system.**
- In the same way we naturally resist eating food that's too much for our systems, **the body cannot digest an intact lactose molecule.**

CHAPTER 5

WHAT HAPPENS WHEN WE INGEST LACTOSE?

Our Inner Highway: The Lymphatic System

I mentioned in the last chapter that the lymphatic system is part of our immune system. The lymphatic system functions as a subset of the immune system, which is the overall defense system of the body. The immune system is called a "system," but it consists of both structures and processes. In contrast, the lymphatic system is made up entirely of biological structures: lymph vessels, lymph nodes, lymphatic fluid, and organs such as the tonsils and spleen.

In this chapter, we'll discuss

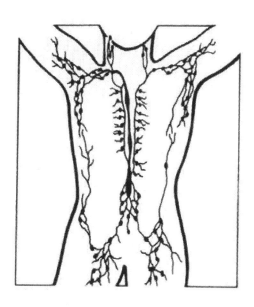

The human lymphatic system, consisting of lymph nodes and lymph vessels (which carry lymphatic fluid).

how the lymphatic system works. Then I'll explain my theory about how lactose is associated with the lymphatic system.

To begin, think of the lymphatic system as an inner highway of your body. The primary function of the lymphatic system is to carry white blood cells (also called leukocytes) around your body.

But what, exactly, do the white blood cells *do*?

The Three Jobs of the Lymphatic System

Simply put, white blood cells travel the body via the *"lymphatic highway."* But what is their purpose in using the highway?

For simplicity's sake, let's take cars out of our highway analogy. Instead, imagine only "working" vehicles on your lymphatic highway. These working vehicles are white blood cells.

There are three types of working vehicles on the lymphatic highway, with three specific jobs:

- **Garbage Truck:** The job of this vehicle is to help remove cellular waste from the body.
- **Emergency Vehicles:** Think fire trucks, ambulances, and police cars. Their job is to heal minor infections anywhere in the body where such infections occur.
- **Military:** Imagine there's an Army truck on your lymphatic highway. That truck is there to bring the best of the best to fight the most serious causes – severe infections or diseases anywhere in your body.

Though they have specific and distinct functions, all three types of vehicles run on the same highway – the lymphatic system. They work together to maintain your overall health.

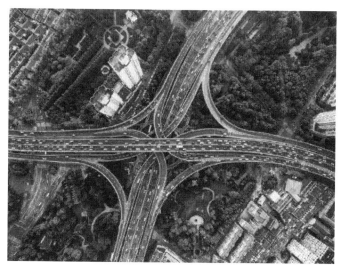

Imagine this highway is your lymphatic system. It takes a lot of "vehicles"
(i.e., white blood cells) to keep your body running smoothly!

Like traffic on a highway, your lymphatic system is in constant motion. It order to keep everything in your body functioning as it should, it's essential that your lymphatic system functions smoothly.

In other words – for you to be healthy, your lymphatic system has to be healthy, too.

Lymph Nodes: Your Body's Filters

Have you ever had swollen lymph nodes? If you have, you know that it's no fun – but those swollen lymph nodes are performing a vital function. When your lymph nodes are swollen, it means your lymphatic system has kicked into high gear to get rid of infection.

Lymph nodes are also filters for the lymphatic system. The job of "garbage truck" lymphocytes (a type of leukocyte – or white blood cell – only found within the lymphatic system) is to clean out the system. All of the "yuck" in cellular waste goes into the lymphatic system and is taken to the lymph nodes, where it's filtered out.

Think of it like the engine in your car. All the particles in motor oil that would keep your car's engine from running smoothly are filtered into the oil filter. The "good oil" goes through and it does the job it's supposed to do.

Your lymph nodes are like six hundred oil filters in your body. It's vital that the filters – your lymph nodes – are able to do their job.

Digesting Lactose

So how does lactose play into this? Conventional science says lactose has no bearing on the lymphatic system. But I believe it does.

As we've already discussed, lactose is a disaccharide. As such, it's a relatively large molecule, because it's composed of two connected molecules. And we know that without the presence of the enzyme lactase, intact lactose cannot be absorbed by the small intestine.

So what happens to that unabsorbed lactose?

In the small intestine, nutrients are separated from waste. When lactase is present and lactose is broken in half, the lactose is hydrolyzed (i.e., broken down by water) into glucose and galactose. Like other nutrients, these glucose and galactose molecules are absorbed through the small intestinal wall. They're then picked up by the bloodstream and taken to a cell that needs a carbohydrate or sugar.

If lactose is *not* hydrolyzed into glucose and galactose, it goes out the bowels as waste. Conventional wisdom says that because a lactose molecule is so large, any lactose that goes out as waste causes the gastrointestinal issues that are classic symptoms of lactose intolerance.

Does *All* Non-Hydrolyzed Lactose Turn Into Waste?

Before I began my lactose-free diet, this was all news to me. I had a vague sense of these basic functions, but I'd given little thought to the specifics.

As I learned in detail about these functions of the body, they made sense to me – for the most part. These functions, as they are conventionally understood, explain why lactose intolerant individuals have gastrointestinal issues. When the body of a lactose intolerant individual tries to eliminate those large, intact lactose molecules, it simply cannot do so without causing pain.

Fair enough. But since I'm not lactose intolerant and I've never had chronic gastrointestinal issues, I was pretty sure something else was going on, too.

I thought about what I'd learned about the lymphatic system. I considered how my symptoms that improved on a lactose free diet were all related to a healthy, functioning lymphatic system.

Because of the dramatic effects on my lymphatic system of removing lactose from my diet, I began to wonder: *what if all the intact lactose isn't going out as waste?*

Could it be, I theorized, that *some of the lactose is making its way into the lymphatic system*? And if so, what effect would it have on our lymphatic highway?

How might lactose impact the three jobs – removing cellular waste, fighting minor infection, and attacking major infections and diseases – which our lymphatic system, when functioning properly, is supposed to do?

Is This the Same as Leaky Gut Syndrome?

When I began exploring these issues, I had the same question. It's worth noting that leaky gut syndrome is not a recognized medical condition. Those who believe in it think it causes chronic inflammation. Leaky gut syndrome, also sometimes called intestinal permeability, is a condition in which – it's believed – toxins and bacteria that affect the overall health of the body leak from the small intestine into other parts of the body. Many who believe in leaky gut syndrome swear by supplements, herbal preparations, or other remedies for resolution of symptoms.

What I'm talking about is similar, but not exactly the same. I don't know if toxins and bacterial leak from the small intestines of some people. And if they do, I don't know if there are outside remedies to fix that problem.

What I *do* believe is that **the one thing that permeates the small intestinal wall and compromises our health is lactose.** I believe that when lactose permeates the small intestinal wall and gets into the lymphatic system, our health is at risk.

Whether or not anything else permeates the small intestinal wall is – in my mind – immaterial. If the lymphatic system isn't compromised – if it's functioning as it's intended to – then it will combat issues like toxins or bacteria that end up somewhere in the body where they're not supposed to be.

Let's look at the root symptom of leaky gut syndrome: a small intestinal wall that's become too elastic. But how did that happen? We can answer that question by asking another one: what is the condition of the lymphatic system? If the lymphatic system is not functioning properly, it cannot combat issues in the small intestine. And the result is an intestinal wall that becomes stretched, possibly allowing toxins and bacteria to leak through.

In my mind, lactose is *always* able to get through. The reason bacteria and toxins might be able to get through, too, is that lactose has done its damage – which, in turn, makes the elasticity of the small intestine even worse.

The system is interconnected. A compromised lymphatic system might make the pancreas inflamed. It might make the kidneys or adrenal glands cease to function properly. It's all a domino effect.

So how do you fix it? You remove the inflammation.

And how do you do that? You remove the lactose.

Lactose-Free Stories: *The Truth About Cats and Dogs*

As we've already discussed, every mammal produces lactase when it is young and its primary food source is its mother's milk. Lactase enables the young mammal to break lactose into glucose and galactose, which a growing mammal's body uses for energy and development.

But animals do not retain the ability to produce lactase. There is no such thing as lactase persistence in animals, because animals have not evolved to have this trait, the way some humans have.

And yet, we give a cat a dish of milk. We feed our dogs ice cream and frozen treats. Many dog and cat foods have milk, cheese, or both as an ingredient.

A cat or dog's immune system works the same way ours does. They have the exact same lymphatic highway as humans, with the exact same three functions: removing cellular waste, fighting minor infection, and fighting major infection and disease.

Is it possible, then, that lactose is making our pets unhealthy? I believe it is. Giving dairy to your dog or cat is, in my opinion, a one-way ticket to the vet.

Cancer is the leading cause of death in dogs over the age of ten (that's seventy in people years). Fifty percent of dogs ten and over develop (and usually die from) cancer. Many might say there is no way to prevent cancer in our pets. But I disagree. I think taking your pet off any food or treat that contains dairy will benefit the pet's health. Will it cure cancer? Perhaps not – but it might prevent your pet from getting cancer in the first place.

When Shelly and I stopped eating dairy, we also looked at our dog's food to see if it contained milk. There is no requirement for pet food packaging to say "CONTAINS MILK," the way human food packaging must. But there is an FDA requirement that pet food packaging must list the food's ingredients.

Before we removed the dairy from our dog's diet, we used to feed him ice cream as a treat. Yummy, I'm sure, but I'll bet he wasn't a fan of the boils he developed as a result. Since he no longer eats dairy, the boils have vanished. In fact, with the exception of regular checkups, he hasn't had to see the vet at all.

It sobers us to remember that the dog we had before this one – another canine with plenty of dairy in his diet – died of lymphoma, which is cancer of the lymph nodes.

We have a cat, too – a twelve-year-old named Cocoa. She used to be a puker. Anyone with a cat who throws up regularly knows what I'm talking about. You're cleaning it off the carpet, sometimes off the furniture. It's gross, but you think it's normal. Cats puke, right? That's just what they do.

Never in my wildest dreams did I think that we were giving Cocoa lactose. We took dairy from the dog's diet but we didn't even think about the cat – and she was still puking.

So here we are, a few months into lactose-free living. The

people are healthy, the dog is healthy – and poor Cocoa is still throwing up. So I checked the ingredients in her food, and sure enough – it contained dairy. We threw it out and found her a dairy-free brand instead. Cocoa hasn't puked since.

A guy I work with overheard me talking about my theory as it relates to humans. I mentioned that I think it applies for pets, too. He said, "I've been taking my dog to the vet for a month now. He keeps scratching himself. He's allergic to everything and they've tried everything, but they can't find anything to help him."

"Do you give your dog treats?" I asked. "What kind of food do you feed him? Have you checked its ingredients list?"

He said he did give treats and that he knew little about what was in the dog's food.

"Look at the treats and the food," I advised. "If there's milk or cheese, find another brand."

He said he'd try it. Two weeks later, he told me his dog had stopped itching.

"It doesn't surprise me," I replied. "It doesn't surprise me at all that that happened."

Lactose-Free Stories: *Mikkel*

Speaking of pets, it's worth mentioning that my brother Mikkel doesn't have any. That's because he's extremely allergic to cats and dogs. In the late 1980s, my parents bought a home in which it was obvious that the previous owners had a cat. The first night we lived there, Mikkel's reaction was so bad my parents had to take him to the emergency room. They were told that he could have died if they hadn't acted as quickly as they did. His face was swollen shut. I'll never forget that.

A few years ago, Mikkel also learned that he's lactose intolerant. He began limiting his lactose intake, but he didn't go completely dairy-free. After I discovered the benefits of lactose-free living – and Mikkel may be forty-five years old but he's still my little brother, so of course I'm allowed to tell him what to do – my brother realized that since he'd started to limit ice cream and had stopped drinking milk, he can spend hours in a house where there's a cat or dog. It used to be just a few minutes, then he'd have to leave or risk having a reaction. But now he can stay for hours with no problems.

Lactose-Free Stories: *Dallas*
Another family member whom I continued to pressure is my twenty-two-year-old stepson Dallas. He was living with us, and Shelly and I had begun talking incessantly about the benefits of lactose-free living. We'd sit out on the patio discussing it like it was the weather.

We finally wore Dallas down, and since December of 2017 he's been lactose-free. It took him a while to get on board – probably because he didn't have any issues other than occasional but severe heartburn. He'd say it felt like his heart was going to burst into flames. The heartburn seemed to be triggered by apple juice (weird, I know) and cheese (not at all surprising to me).

Since he started eating a lactose-free diet, Dallas has had zero issues with heartburn. He tried apple juice one day and everything was fine – no heartburn.

He said, "I can't believe I can drink apple juice and nothing happens."

"Sure you can," I told him. "Just don't go back to the cheese."

Other than the heartburn, Dallas was (and still is) as healthy as they come. But he agrees with me now. He knows there's something to this.

Chris's Lactose-Free Takeaways

The lymphatic system is the key to our health. In learning about this system, I discovered:

- The **lymphatic system is much like a highway,** and the vehicles (lymphocytes) that run on it perform vital tasks that keep the body healthy.
- A thriving, functional lymphatic system **clears out cellular waste, attacks minor infections, and fights major diseases** in the body.
- My theory is that **large, intact lactose molecules clog the lymphatic system** and prevent it from doing its jobs.

CHAPTER 6

THE LYMPHATIC TRAFFIC JAM

My Theory

I've mentioned this already, but it bears repeating: I'm not a scientist or a doctor. I came up with this theory completely on my own. I would be thrilled to see this theory investigated by the scientific community, but to my knowledge no such studies exist at this time.

Building on what we talked about in the last chapter, I began to wonder: *what if some of the intact lactose, instead of leaving the body as waste, passes through the small intestinal wall?*

My theory is that it does. I believe at least some of the large, intact lactose molecules hitch a ride to a cell in the body that has signaled it needs a carbohydrate or a sugar.

Remember that quadruple cheeseburger we talked about? For a cell, the intact lactose molecule is like that. It's simply too big for the cell to use.

So what does the cell do with it? Exactly what you'd do with a rock-solid quadruple cheeseburger: the cell throws the lactose in the trash and waits for something more palatable to come along.

And for cells, where is that trash?

It's the lymphatic system.

Clogging the Lymphatic Filter

Keep in mind that the lymphatic system is a filtration system. The system is filled with lymphocytes that do three jobs: kill infections, combat invaders anywhere they're found in the body, and move cellular waste to organs such as the kidneys and lungs, which continue the process of expelling cellular waste from the body.

My belief is that when the lymphatic system is clogged with lactose, the lymphocytes cannot do their jobs. They're simply not suited to catching something as big as a lactose molecule and eliminating it quickly.

The bottom line is, the system is unable to take out this type of garbage.

The Lymphatic Traffic Jam

So what happens when the lymphatic system has too much lactose in it? Instead of doing their jobs, the lymphocytes are sitting in a traffic jam.

The lymphocytes are supposed to be fighting the flu or fighting cancer. Their job is to fight whatever is ailing the body. But in a system clogged with lactose, the lymphocytes are not getting where they need to be quickly enough.

Lactose backs up our lymphatic system. This creates a traffic jam, preventing the lymphocytes – essentially, the primary mechanisms of health in our bodies – from doing their job.

In the way it's structured, the lymphatic system is similar to the circulatory system. Just as the veins and arteries through which blood moves are huge compared to capillaries, lymph vessels entering the lymph nodes are much bigger than the vessels going out. The systems work the same way: big pipes turn into small pipes that turn into even smaller pipes.

It's also like our system of roadways: big highways turn into smaller highways, turn into backstreets, turn into alleys.

And in any of these systems, congestion is congestion. A traffic jam is going to cause the system to come to a standstill.

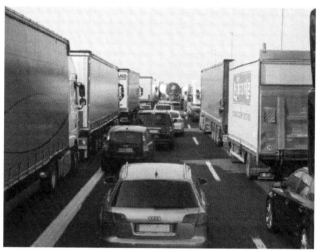

A congested lymphatic system looks like this. What emergency vehicle could make it through?

Call in the Troops!

Let's look at an example. Say a cell mutates and becomes cancerous. The lymphatic system sends its best lymphocytes – the "Navy Seals of the immune system" – to destroy it.

Now imagine an eighteen-wheeler is broken down in the middle of the highway that those Navy Seals were on, trying to get to the cancer threat. And then maybe another truck slams into the back of the first one. These trucks represent huge lactose molecules which are jamming the lymphatic system. And they're not going anywhere anytime soon. Before you know it, you've got an enormous a traffic jam on your hands. The garbage truck is at a standstill next to you, and so are the Navy Seals. A helicopter can't even take off. Nothing can get where it needs to be.

Lymphocytes are supposed to be swapped out every three days. The system only sends the best of the best to take out a perceived threat of this magnitude. But when there's a lymphatic traffic jam, these exceptional lymphocytes cannot quickly get where they're needed most.

Cells within every person's body have the ability to mutate and become cancerous. You can't "catch" cancer. When a cell mutates into cancer, the lymphatic system is supposed to smash it immediately. But when the lymphatic system is compromised, its ability to deal with cancerous cells is compromised, too.

Remember how we talked about Ponce de Leon's "Fountain of Youth"? I think it's interesting to note that in many Native American languages, there isn't a word for cancer. They didn't need that word, because before Europeans arrived, they never had anything like cancer. They didn't have cancer until their immune systems were weakened by the adoption of a typically European, dairy-heavy diet.

Here's another example. Let's say an allergen has entered the body through nose. A crowd of lymphocytes comes to the rescue. If the lymphatic system is working as designed, when your body recognizes that it needs help, assistance arrives immediately. But when the lymphatic system is compromised, it's the immediateness that's compromised. The lymphocytes might still get there, but not as quickly. The speed at which the lymphocytes are getting around the body, how fast and how healthy they are when they get where they're needed, is also being compromised.

Clearing Out the Traffic Jam

When we remove lactose from our diets, our lymphatic system

clears itself out. This can take some time, but eventually the system will start functioning as it was originally intended to. Nothing will block the way of the lymphocytes getting where they need to be in order to do their jobs.

As the system clears out, the body will address its most pressing issues one by one. For some individuals it might be congestion. For others, it could be asthma or allergies – or any number of other concerns. There's no way to know how a particular body (human or pet) will react, except to give lactose-free living a try.

You know that feeling when you think you're getting sick? You get that tickle. You get that itch. You get that and you think – okay, I know tomorrow is going to be a rough day.

On a lactose-free diet, you might still get that initial feeling. But because your lymphatic system is clear, because your lymphocytes can arrive quickly to address the problem – that "rough day" never comes.

There is one result that I've noticed is universal among everyone I've talked to who has adopted a lactose-free lifestyle:

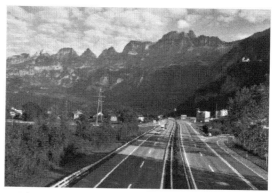

It's a smooth ride on this gorgeous, unclogged highway.

when the lymphatic system becomes clean and pure, when it gets back to its original state and is working as it was designed, that's clarity.

Everyone I've talked to who removed lactose from their diet has talked about mental clarity. I fully believe this occurs because the lymphatic system is no longer being clogged by lactose.

Your Immune System is in Control

The immune system – of which the lymphatic system plays a key role – is in control of everything in the body. The immune system is the "backbone" of a healthy body.

Speaking of bones – most of us have been taught that we get strong bones and longevity from drinking milk. But this isn't true. You get strong bones and longevity from having a healthy immune system.

And how do you achieve a healthy immune system? It's all based on your dietary choices.

And when it comes to your diet, you're in the driver's seat.

Lactose-Free Stories: *Marlene*

I love to tell the story of my mother's journey to lactose-free living, because her transformation has been truly extraordinary.

My mom's name is Marlene. She's eighty years old. Her heritage is one hundred percent Norwegian. Some years ago, she had a stroke, and afterward, my dad attended to her daily needs. Then, about two years ago, my parents moved into my sister's house in Chicago, because my dad's health was deteriorating, too. Basically, he could no longer take care of both himself and my mom.

Soon after my parents moved into my sister's home, my mom was diagnosed with Parkinson's. At the time, I didn't converse with her very often. It was hard…I wanted to speak with her, but she didn't seem to understand what I said on the phone, and she didn't say much in response.

What I *did* do was talk to my dad. This was in early 2017, not long after I'd begun my lactose-free lifestyle.

"Dad," I said. "I think a dairy-free diet might help you and

Mom. What I'm going through and what I'm seeing in all the other people who have taken dairy out of their diets – you can't tell me it's not going to help you guys too. Whether it's a wart or Parkinson's," I told him, "…or anything in between…honestly, there's nothing that I don't think this is going help with."

My parents listened to me and adopted a partially dairy-free diet. They bought almond milk and began to eat more peanut butter. They'd never been big cheese eaters, so that wasn't an issue, but they were still using butter. Additionally, my dad loved milk chocolate and wasn't willing to give it up.

On a diet of limited dairy, they were both doing fine, but there were no enormous improvements in their health. Mom improved slightly – everybody in the family could see the slight improvements – but it was nothing dramatic.

When I talked to my dad, occasionally he'd hand the phone to Mom. We'd have our one-minute conversation; that's all she could manage. I'd tell her she should try to eat as little dairy as she possibly could. My dad said she seemed to understand this. But because she wasn't the one buying the food or making the meals, it was hard for her to be 100% dairy-free,

In August of 2017, I saw my parents for the first time in a number of months. The family always gathers in August to remember my oldest brother, Chinny, who passed away of his second heart attack at age fifty-six. We have an annual golf tournament in memory of Chinny. In 2017 we had the tournament in the town where Chinny raised his family.

That's where I got to sit down and spend some time with my mom. I listened to her talk. I told her how great she's doing and how much better she sounds.

"You know," I told her. "This is something you need to stick with. You need to get really serious about eating a completely dairy-free diet."

I'm a lucky son in that I have a mom who listens to me simply because I'm her son. Plus, she could see the great results I was getting. From that point on, she was convinced. She talked with my sister about it and asked her to make sure nothing that she (Mom) ate had dairy in it. Mom has been eating 100% lactose-free ever since that family gathering in August of 2017.

So, of course, the big question is – how has her health changed?

In a word: dramatically. At the three-month mark of being 100% lactose-free, she was able to have an engaging and mean-ingful phone conversation. She was no longer falling into walls. She could go up and down the stairs unassisted. She still had Parkinson's – she still wasn't the self she'd been before the Par-kinson's – but she was getting so much better.

When I saw her at Christmas, she said – as many others have – that the mental clarity was the biggest change. Before going completely lactose-free, she couldn't even remember her own name. Now she could handily beat me in a game of cribbage!

She lost weight, and that made her really happy. "I weigh 146 pounds," she said at Christmas. "I haven't been in my 140s for twenty years." Nowadays, she weighs 137 and she's wearing skinny jeans. She was never an obese woman, but when we kids were growing up, she was always worried about her weight. She'd been on every fad diet in existence, but nothing worked – she'd never lose more than ten pounds. She's lost thirty pounds now, and if you asked her what she's most happy about, it would be her weight.

Her balance is so good, she can bend over at the waist and

pick up a dime between her feet. This is a woman who, previously, couldn't stand up without tipping into a wall.

She saw her neurologist and passed every memory test the doctor put in front of her. These were tests she'd failed just a few months before.

She's had high cholesterol for a long time but she's never been able to take medication for it. Not long ago, I took her to visit the doctor in Arizona that she'd seen before moving to Chicago. She asked him if he remembered her.

"Of course, I remember you," he said. "I remember that you have high cholesterol and you can't take any medication for it."

"Her cholesterol will be better now," I assured him.

"We'll see about that," he replied

"She's taken lactose out of her diet," I went on. "That's the only thing she's changed. And all of her health benefits have skyrocketed. I guarantee you, doctor – her cholesterol is going to be down as well."

They drew blood and ran the tests. Her cholesterol was lower by eighty points, all of it LDL (the "bad" cholesterol).

Sadly, my dad passed away in December of 2017. Since then, my mom has come out to Arizona several times and is now planning to move back to Arizona. She's devastated to have lost my dad, of course, but her mental health improvements are extraordinary. As time goes on, I see her continually get brighter and brighter.

Her joint pain has disappeared. She told me that used to cry herself to sleep because she knew that after Dad died, no one would be there to help her get out of bed. She used to wake up in the middle of night and her ankles would hurt, her elbow would hurt, her shoulder would hurt – everything. Now she wakes up feeling fine. She just flips over and rolls out of bed.

She's been practicing getting on her hands and knees on the floor, then rising to standing from that position. She's doing that because she doesn't want to be someone who has "fallen and can't get up."

She has eight adult children. Every one of us believes she could live independently. We think she can do almost everything on her own. She wants to live by herself and we're going to try to make that happen.

As to the "why" of this – my siblings are on the fence. Some of them believe it's her medication – even though she's now taking less than half the medication she was before she went lactose-free. She's down to nine pills a day – she had been taking twenty-one pills daily. She's been weaned off everything else.

My opinion is that it's not the medication; it's her body fixing itself. Her immune system now does what it's intended to do.

Not long ago, I took her to the doctor to see what he thought of her cholesterol drop. He told her all her numbers were good except for her high cholesterol. I could tell he was about to give her a high cholesterol lecture, so I said, "Is an eighty point drop in a matter of eight months typical? All of it LDL?"

His answer was, "No." I went on to remind him about her lactose-free diet.

I asked him to be her permanent doctor, now that she's back in Arizona. She had a follow-up with him in August. The doctor has permitted her to drop another four pills a day; these were for blood pressure and he said they were no longer necessary. Doing the math, she's taking *4,380* less pills a year than she'd been taking twelve months earlier!

These days, my mom is adamant about her diet. She'll eat anything else – but she will *not* put lactose in her body.

Lactose-Free Stories: *Beth*

My sister Beth is in her late fifties and, like the rest of the family, is of German and Norwegian descent. Shortly after our mom began eating a 100% lactose-free diet, Beth adopted the lactose-free lifestyle, too. The reasons were obvious to her by then. Beth is the sister with whom our parents lived in Chicago, and she was the one who managed Mom's neurological appointments and other doctor visits. It's crystal-clear to Beth how much better Mom is now that she eats no dairy.

Beth called me last winter to tell me she's now lactose-free, because of our mother's extraordinary results.

"That's great," I said. "I'm so happy to hear it, Beth."

"I have to tell you," she went on. "The flu just went through our household. Everyone in the household got it. Everyone who came over to the house got it. Every single person was bedridden, except for two people: Mom and me."

So, the two people whose immune systems were able to fight off the flu that no one else's system could combat? Those two people are also the only two lactose-free people in the house.

It wasn't always this way. Beth used to have blocks of cheese in kitchen drawers – I kid you not. And I bet there were another fifty pounds of cheese in her refrigerator. She would have been one of the last people I'd have expected to give up dairy completely.

Honestly, Beth being lactose-free is incredible. She gives me hope for everybody!

Chris's Lactose-Free Takeaways

In thinking of the lymphatic system as a highway, I've come to believe that:

- **Intact lactose molecules jam the "lymphatic highway"** and prevent lymphocytes from doing their jobs.
- When the lymphatic system is **working as designed, health and clarity are the result.**
- **These results are within the reach of everyone,** because they are controlled by the choice to remove lactose from one's diet.

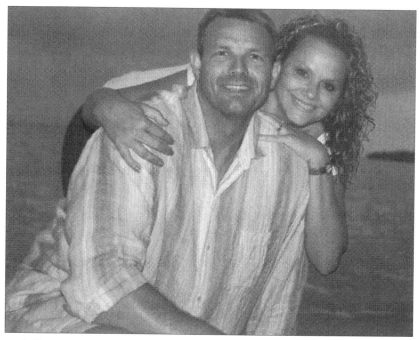

Shelly and me in 2014, a few years before we discovered lactose-free living.

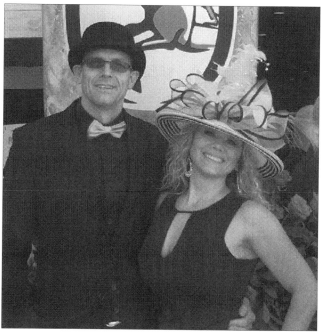

What a difference a new lifestyle makes! Shelly and me at the Kentucky Derby, 2017.

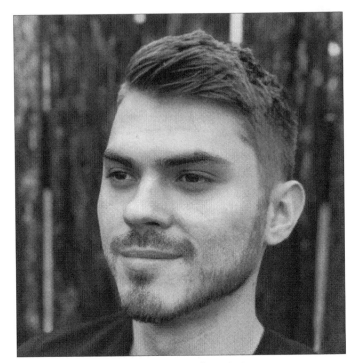

Quentin, September 2018.

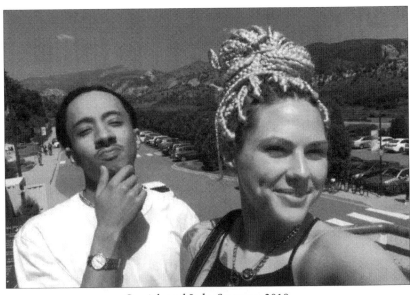

Garrick and Jade, Summer 2018.

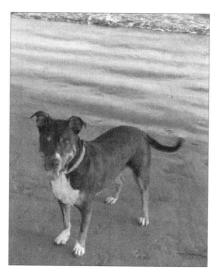

Our lactose-free dog, Boss – having fun and looking good on the beach in 2017.

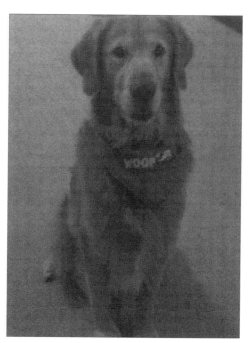

Our previous dog. My heart breaks when I read comments about him on Shelly's Facebook page. From a friend: "I remember the first time he came to the house. He fell in love with cheese! Precious boy!" Shelly's response: "He sure did love cheese. Any time he would hear the plastic come off the cheese, he would be right there waiting to get his slice. He was such a good dog!"

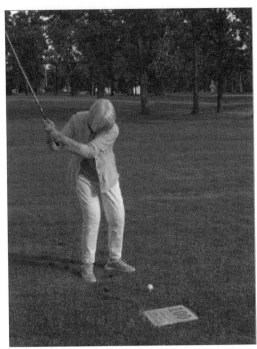

My mother, Marlene, golfing at age eighty. This is at our family golf tournament, Summer 2018.

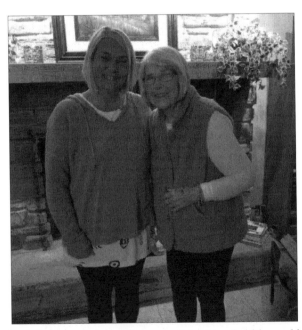

My sister, Beth, and our mother, Marlene – both looking healthy and happy, living a lactose-free lifestyle in 2018.

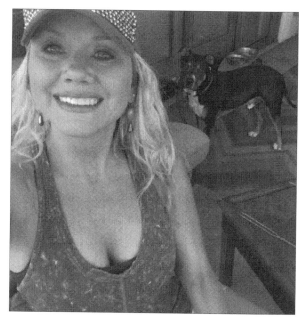

Shelly, with our dog, Boss, in the background, 2018.

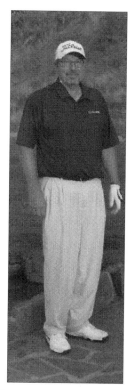

My brother, Luke – trim, fit, and heart-healthy in 2017.

CHAPTER 7

PROVING IT TO MYSELF: VISITING THE MAYO CLINIC

Discovery is Exciting, but Proof is Everything

As I'm sure you can imagine, I was pretty excited to have come up with this theory. My results, as well as the results for others I knew who had eliminated lactose from their diets, was astounding.

I told everyone I knew about it. I made a slide presentation, and whenever I had the opportunity, I opened my laptop and showed the slides anyone who would listen to me.

I even went so far as setting up an appointment with a patent attorney. I knew I had nothing to patent (What was I going to patent? A theory?), but still, I thought the attorney could give me some insight into how I could get the word out widely about what I think lactose does to the body. She was intrigued but had few suggestions from a legal perspective.

I could continue spreading the word one person at a time, but I knew that a scientific study would be the best way to widely distribute this information. To the best of my knowledge, no such study has been done to date.

Something amazing had occurred – no doubt about it – but now I faced another dilemma: how could I get the scientific and/ or medical community on board?

The Mayo Clinic

In trying to solve that dilemma, I came across an intriguing possibility: the Mayo Clinic. Most people know about the not-for-profit Mayo Clinic based in Rochester, Minnesota. The facility in Rochester, in addition to having a long and outstanding history of providing inpatient and outpatient care for people with a variety of illnesses, is also a top-notch research facility. What's not as commonly known is that Mayo also operates a smaller hospital in Phoenix.

It was to the Phoenix facility that I inquired. Soon thereafter, I was admitted into the Mayo Clinic's Consultative Medicine Program. I was accepted into the program for two reasons: because of my branchial cleft fistulas and because my family has such a high risk of death via heart disease at an early age.

Full disclosure: I didn't enter the program in order to get a diagnosis and subsequent treatment plan. I knew I was 100% healthy. What I wanted was for the Mayo doctors to show me how healthy I actually *was* – and, maybe, for some of them to become intrigued by my theory.

My First Appointment

The first time I went to the Mayo facility in Phoenix, I'd been eating a lactose-free diet for eleven months. I was handed a questionnaire to fill out, with approximately forty questions on it.

I took a seat and got to work. It was astounding. For nineteen of the listed issues, I checked "No, I don't have this, but yes, I used to."

It was like a "before" and "after" checklist of giving up dairy. Nearly half of the items the questionnaire asked me about had been resolved by eliminating dairy from my diet.

Seeing the Cardiologists

Because of my family history of heart attacks, I saw two different cardiologists. They did a blood workup, an EKG, and other tests. They had me do a stress test on a treadmill.

We talked about heart attacks, and this is what one of the cardiologists said: "To have a heart attack, you've got to have somewhere around 80% or 90% blockage. But do you know why one person with that level of blockage has a heart attack while another with the same level doesn't?"

I told him that I did not know.

"Inflammation," he told me. "The one that has inflammation is going to have the heart attack."

To test the inflammation in the body, the doctors use a C-Reactive Protein High Sensitivity Test. C-Reactive Protein is a substance produced by the liver that increases in the presence of inflammation. According to the C-Reactive Protein High Sensitivity Test, my inflammation is zero.

Other than minor carotid plaque buildup, all of my numbers came back great. Nonetheless, after examining me, one of the cardiologists recommended that I go on a statin medication just as a precaution, given of my family history. I politely turned him down, promising to check my blood pressure at home and stay on top of getting regular blood workups.

When the second cardiologist examined me, his take was a bit different.

"You know," he told me. "I'm a huge fan of statins. They're so effective for so many people, I would put them in the water if I could."

He went on, "I can't believe I'm saying this to you. Even with your history of heart disease, high cholesterol, and everything else you've listed, I – the doctor who would put statins in the water if I could – can't justify prescribing a statin to you. That's how good your numbers are."

All Those Doctors

All in all, I saw seven different medical providers (physicians or physician's assistants) at the Mayo, on five separate occasions that took place in December 2017 through February 2018. Some of the providers wanted to know about my branchial cleft fistulas. Others (like the two mentioned above) evaluated my cardiovascular system. Some were focused on my overall health.

I told each of them about my lactose-free diet. They were all clear on the fact that I attribute my great health to eliminating lactose from my system.

So what did they think? Well, they were all pleasant and encouraging. They all told me that clearly I was doing something right, and since it was working for me, I should keep it up.

None of them denied that my lactose-free lifestyle was the reason for my overall great health. But none confirmed it, either.

Meeting Dr. Snyder

Dr. Snyder was one of the final doctors I saw at the Mayo Clinic. He evaluated my overall health and looked at the reports from the other medical providers I'd seen at the Clinic. We talked about ***integrative medicine*** – that is, taking a holistic approach by combining evidence-based alternative and complementary medicine with traditional western medicine.

I'll admit it – I talked a lot during this interview. I told Dr. Snyder my theory about lactose clogging the lymphatic system. I told him about my mother's Parkinson's. I explained how much better she's doing since eliminating dairy completely from her diet. I told him about the others, too – Quentin and Dallas, Garrick and Jade, and everyone else I knew who'd stopped eating dairy products and had experienced significant improvements to their health.

"That is an amazing story," Dr. Snyder said. "Maybe you should write a book!"

In his report on my health, Dr. Snyder called me an **"N of 1."** I didn't know what that meant, so I looked it up. I learned that "N of 1" refers to a clinical trial that only studies one person. Although I disagree with the doctor – I'm an N of *many*, when you consider all the people I know who have given up dairy – I found the term intriguing.

This is why I used a variant of it for the title of this book. I may be an "N of 1" in Dr. Snyder's eyes – but if I am, it's because it's been the **eNd** of one lifestyle and the beginning of a fantastic new one.

Can Someone Live This Lifestyle and Stay Healthy?

Dr. Snyder and I talked in depth about what I eat. He expressed concern about me following a diet completely free of dairy products. He worried about keeping up a healthy nutritional lifestyle without all of the foods that contain lactose.

He asked me, "Can you live healthfully without dairy?"

"I believe you can," I told him. "I believe that if you eliminate lactose, you can eat whatever you want and your body will be able to use it because your lymphatic system will be functioning properly."

"Well, keep up the good work," Dr. Snyder said. "It will be interesting to see how this evolves over time."

Lactose-Free Stories: *Shelly*

I've saved the story of Shelly, my wife, for a bit later in this book, because it's more complicated than the stories of others we've already talked about.

Shelly is forty-two years old. She's white, but she's not sure of her specific heritage. She thinks she might have a small bit of Native American heritage, but she's not sure about that. We've been married for eight years.

As I mentioned early, Shelly is overall healthy. But she does have an autoimmune disorder. It's called lymphocytic colitis. Symptoms include swelling and digestion issues. Because of her disorder, she's spent a lot of years looking for ways to improve her health. I remember years ago she did a green smoothie cleanse. It was supposed to be for ten days, but she did twenty. Another time she went to Thailand and lived on nothing but grapes for weeks on end.

These things temporarily helped Shelly feel better – which, in retrospect, doesn't surprise me. When you're doing a cleanse or eating very little, your body isn't spending all its time digesting food. There are two things the body can't do at the same time: repair itself and digest food. If a person is constantly eating, the body must focus on digestion. This leaves few resources available for doing repair work. When it's digesting, the body is not in a mode of regeneration.

When we fast, the body isn't focused on digestion. This gives the body the ability to regenerate and mend itself. That's what was going on with Shelly's cleanses and grape fasts.

Also – and this is key – when you remove just about everything from your diet, one of those things is sure to be dairy. In my opinion, nothing else involved in a cleanse – removing carbs, meat, caffeine, alcohol, any of that – matters much. It's the removal of dairy from the diet, allowing the body to begin healing because the lymphatic system is no longer clogged with lactose, that makes a difference.

But – as anyone who's done a cleanse will attest – extreme dietary changes are not sustainable long-term. Nor are they meant to be. They help, but if you finish the cleanse (or return from your trip to Thailand) and resume your old habits, things will go back to what they were before.

Shelly knows this. She works hard to eat a healthy diet every day. Currently, she's vegan – so, of course, she eats no dairy. There are a lot of other things she doesn't eat, either – and she feels better eating this way. Also, just as importantly, she feels she can maintain this dietary lifestyle long-term.

I had high hopes when we began our dairy-free diet (which evolved into a vegan diet for Shelly) that her lymphocytic colitis would go away. She lost about twenty-five pounds and has had zero infections since removing lactose from her diet. Everything as far as her immune health is perfect. But – though her immune system is functioning at 100% – Shelly still has lymphocytic colitis.

Why? We're not sure, but I believe it's because Shelly's main issue is autoimmune. So in her system, the good is fighting the bad (which explains her weight loss, lack of infections, and other improvements) – but at the same time, the good is still fighting the good. This is the exact definition of an autoimmune disease: the immune system can't tell the difference between a "good" cell and a "bad" cell, so it attacks them both. It's like the Army fighting the Navy or the Marines fighting the Air Force.

So in Shelly's system, the good is still fighting the good, which is why her lymphocytic colitis remains. There are other diseases that behave similarly: rheumatoid arthritis, psoriasis – any autoimmune disorder. I think that even if your immune system is perfectly healthy (i.e., you're not clogging it with lactose), it isn't easy to retrain the system to know what's good and what's bad.

Shelly also had EPI (endocrine pancreatic insufficiency), which means her pancreas wasn't producing the enzyme that separates fats and proteins. Her body was not breaking down fat at all. This was agonizing for her, but I'm happy to report that at this point, her pancreas is functioning better than it used to. In my opinion, this is solely due to the removal of lactose from her diet. Her pancreas is not perfect, but it's producing the enzyme again.

My wife believes in the benefits of a lactose-free diet. She feels much better eating no dairy. But it's hard for her to become as enthused about it as I am because she still suffers with lymphocytic colitis. This is what keeps her from talking to anyone and everyone she meets about it, the way I do.

I wish I had better news for folks out there with an autoimmune disorder. For me, this is yet another reason why thorough research is desperately needed. Perhaps research scientists would be able to get to the bottom of this. Perhaps they could find a way to address the connection between a lactose-free diet and autoimmune disorders.

Chris's Lactose-Free Takeaways

I learned a lot during my visits to the Mayo Clinic, including:

- Completing a checklist of conditions that I used to have but no longer do was like **making a checklist of before and after beginning a lactose-free diet.**

- Many cardiologists are firm believers in statin drugs, but **when an immune system is as healthy as mine, statin drugs are not needed.**
- **Thorough scientific and medical research is needed** into how lactose affects the immune system.

CHAPTER 8

GIVE UP DAIRY? REALLY?

About Now, You Might Be Wondering…

"*…What* am I getting myself into?"

I understand. Giving up dairy might sound like a daunting prospect. But if you've read this far, I hope you're considering a lactose-free diet.

If you are, maybe you have a few questions. Based on conversations I've had with others on this topic, I'd guess you'd like to know:

- How can I live a lactose-free lifestyle when lactose is in so much stuff?
- How can I give up the foods I love? What will I eat instead?
- Can I take lactose out of my diet and still be healthy nutrition-wise?

Trust me – I get it. When I started this process, I had those same questions. I've had to make this lifestyle change without much guidance – but in this chapter, we'll discuss what I've learned about eating lactose-free, and I'll provide some tips to help you get started.

Begin With the Labels

Whatever your politics, I think we can all agree that sometimes it seems like our government is working against us. But I'm happy to report that when it comes to lactose-free living, the U.S. government is actually here to help! Since 2004, there has been a federal law on the books called the Food Allergen Labeling and Consumer Protection Act (FALCPA). The goal of FALCPA is to ensure that labeling of packaged food is clear, easy to read, and simple to understand. The law was proposed and passed to benefit the millions of Americans with food allergies. Whether you have a food allergy or not, FALCPA is good news for anyone concerned with the nutritional value of food products.

FALCPA went into effect on January 1, 2006. Because of FALCPA, any packaged food containing milk (among other allergens, like gluten or soy) has to say so. It's pretty simple, really. If it says "CONTAINS MILK," that means the product contains lactose. Here's an example:

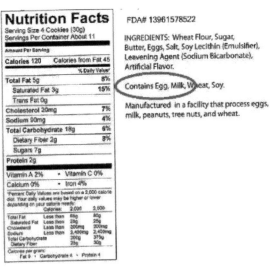

A typical food label

What About Traces?

Some labels say the product may contain "traces" of milk (or other foods). Sometimes it says the product was "processed in a facility that also processes" milk.

Both of these statements mean essentially the same thing: the product was processed in a facility where, for example, the same rollers are used for a bread containing milk as an ingredient as for a batch of dairy-free bread.

In these cases, milk is not one of the ingredients in the finished product. But the product is rolled over the same equipment as the facility uses for rolling products containing milk.

I personally am fine eating such products. I think it would be very difficult to eat only packaged foods that come from completely milk-free facilities. But you can certainly try! If you go this route, a health food store might be a good place to shop.

Dining Out

Like most of us, I love to eat out. There's nothing more pleasurable than a great meal with wonderful company, enjoyed in an establishment with friendly service and a winning atmosphere.

But what if you're trying to eat lactose-free? When you eat out, how will you know what they're putting in your food?

The good news is, many restaurants now offer an allergen menu. If you know the name of the restaurant where you're planning to go, you can look up the allergen menu before you even get there. If you're making a decision on the fly, your smartphone lets you to check this information. This allows you to enter the restaurant prepared.

Even if no allergen menu is available, you can ask your server. People with food allergies do this whenever they go out. It becomes second-nature to them; most people with food allergies never hesitate to get the details about what's on their plate before they dig in. They know what to look for on a menu – and they know that if they want to order anything elaborate, they'll need to ask the server specifically how it's prepared.

If you're uncertain, there are sure-bet foods at almost every restaurant:

- Salads (ask for no cheese on top, choose a dairy-free dressing, and, just to be safe, ask to have the dressing served on the side)
- Fruit
- Plain pasta or potatoes (make sure you request no butter, cheese, sour cream, or other dairy topping)
- Grilled meat, chicken, or fish

If you're having Mexican, go ahead and order that fresh guacamole – there's nothing more satisfying, and you can be assured in pretty much any restaurant that they won't have added dairy to their guacamole.

The Options Are Limitless!

I know that at first glance, the idea of eating zero dairy might seem daunting or even depressing. How can you eat a satisfactory, tasty diet without milk, butter, or ice cream?

"I could never," you might be saying, "never in a million years live without cheese."

But the reality is – yes, you can. There are dairy-free products in every grocery store. Many grocers carry dairy-free sour cream, ice cream – anything, and it tastes awesome.

You can eat a burger – just not a cheeseburger. Eat a bacon-avocado burger if you want – just skip the cheese, and make sure the bun is dairy-free.

Here's something that I think needs to be stated: ***eggs are not dairy.*** Eggs are often grouped with dairy – probably because they both come from a farm – but eggs from a chicken have no relation to milk products from a cow or other mammal. On a lactose-free diet, you can enjoy eggs freely.

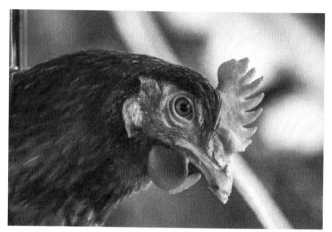

She might live on a farm, the same as a cow does.
But there the similarity ends.

What about baked goods and treats? You can make your own, using a butter substitute. Or you can find dairy-free packaged ones in the store. Want a surprise? Here's one: Nutter Butter cookies don't have lactose. Just stay away from the fudge-striped variety – on the package, you'll see that it says "CONTAINS MILK."

Love butter? I Can't Believe It's Not Butter Vegan tastes just like it. There are also other brands, like Earth Balance and Smart Balance, that spread well and taste delicious.

If you like to cook and you need ideas, there are tons of cookbooks and websites with recipes. Do a search for "dairy free recipes" – or you can even look for something specific, like how to make your own dairy-free cheese substitutes. You'll be amazed at all the possibilities that crop up!

What Will I Feed My Kids?

It might seem difficult to get your kids to adopt a lactose-free diet. As I mentioned in Chapter 2, my own young son eats mostly dairy-free, but it can be tough when our kids spend time with other kids and the food choices all seem to include milk or cheese.

My advice is to simply do the best you can. At home, your kids can drink a plant-based milk and you can make dairy-free meals. You can even get them involved in the meal planning and cooking.

People with lactose intolerant kids or kids with dairy allergies learn to adapt recipes. They alert teachers and school staff, other parents, and caregivers about their child's diet, in anticipation of those times when the child is eating away from home. They supply their children with portable, dairy-free snacks – that way, even if there are no dairy-free options available, their children will have something to eat.

You can do the same. It takes time and perseverance, but it's doable.

Don't We Need Vitamin D and Calcium From Cow's Milk?

As we talked about earlier, the first people to eat dairy probably did so because it was a simple, plentiful food source with a continually replenishing supply (as long as people fed and cared for their cows or goats). But another benefit that was eventually discovered is that milk contains Vitamin D, which is essential for the absorption of calcium. This was especially important in climates where people did not see much sunlight – because sunlight is a natural, non-food source of Vitamin D.

These days, very few people on the planet live in areas where there's little-to-no sunlight. As long as you're spending time outdoors, even with sunscreen (which I certainly advocate using), most people get sufficient Vitamin D from the sun.

If you're unable to spend much time outdoors, there are numerous non-dairy foods that contain Vitamin D: egg yolks, salmon, and trout, to name a few. Many cereals and other packaged foods are fortified with Vitamin D. If you feel you're not getting enough Vitamin D from the sun or from your lactose-free diet, you can always take a non-dairy-based Vitamin D supplement.

What about calcium? It's key to great bone health – but again, there are plenty of sources of calcium besides milk. Did you know that, serving for serving, almond milk contains twice as much calcium as cow's milk? And there are many other excellent sources of calcium – leafy greens, canned fish, and oranges, to name a few.

Almond Milk Doesn't Taste Like "Real" Milk

This is an understandable concern. If you're been drinking milk from a cow or other animal all your life, it might be hard to envision adapting to a plant-based substitute like almond, soy, cashew, or coconut milk.

But I'd like you think about this all-too-common scenario: imagine you go into a restaurant and order a Dr. Pepper. Your server puts the glass on the table and you take a sip – and you almost spit it out.

You think – whoa, that's *not* Dr. Pepper. That tastes terrible.

But it's not terrible. What happened is something that many of us have experienced: you expected to taste Dr. Pepper (or Diet Coke or root beer or something else you ordered that's the same color as Dr. Pepper) but you didn't get what you expected, because your server brought you a Coke.

And it's not terrible. It's just Coke. Does Coke taste terrible? No, but it doesn't taste like Dr. Pepper.

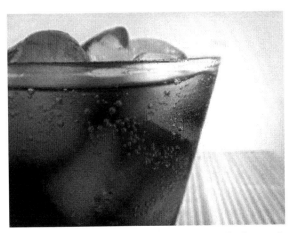

Coke or Dr. Pepper? It's impossible to tell just by how it looks.

It's the same with plant-based milks. If you expect to drink a glass of cow's milk and you take a sip of a plant-based milk, you're in for a rude awakening. But if you pick up a glass of almond milk knowing that's what you're drinking, it's just almond milk. It doesn't taste like cow's milk, but because you're not expecting cow's milk, it tastes fine. Delicious, in fact!

Note: If you're in a coffee shop, you might need to ask for a plant-based milk. Many coffee shops carry it, but it's not always sitting on the counter the way cow's milk or half-and-half is.

Can't I Just Take Lactase Enzyme Pills?

You may have seen these in stores. These supplements are the enzyme lactase in pill form. They're often marketed to lactose intolerant individuals as a way for such individuals to eat dairy without suffering gastrointestinal problems.

I personally don't recommend using these supplements. Did you know that "lactose-free milk" is actually cow's milk with the enzyme lactase added to it? I would never knowingly ingest that. Some users of these supplements report that they work like a charm, while others say they're ineffective or cause unwanted side effects.

But if you simply must eat something containing lactose, I believe it can only benefit you if any lactose you ingest actually breaks down because of using the supplement. Individual results from these products vary, so whether or not to try this method is something you'll have to decide for yourself.

What About Lactose in Medications?

One often-overlooked source of lactose is medications – both prescription and over-the-counter. Lactose is used by the pharmaceutical industry as a bonder. It holds tablets together.

Some allergy medicines, for example, contain a high percentage of lactose. It's ironic. We take allergy pills because our bodies are congested. We believe our bodies can't fight off congestion without medication. But if the medication itself contains lactose, then the medication may be alleviating some of our symptoms – but at the same time, it's exacerbating the problem.

So what can you do? My suggestion should be obvious by now: adopt a lactose-free diet – and over time, evaluate whether you still need all those pills. You might be surprised to discover what you can live without!

A Word on Weight Loss

As you've probably noted from the stories in this book, pretty much everyone who adopts a lactose-free diet loses weight. I can understand why this aspect of lactose-free living might be appealing.

Carrying extra body weight is an all-too-common struggle. In the U.S., two-thirds of adults and one out of every six children aged two through nineteen are overweight or obese. Besides slowing us down physically, being overweight or obese is linked to heart disease, diabetes, cancer, and many other illnesses.

So how does lactose-free living make a difference? Besides helping you eat better quality food, ***the most important reason a lactose-free diet helps you lose weight is because your lymphatic system is functioning properly.*** This means your body is more efficiently using the calories and fuel you're providing to it, in the form of food.

Some people who have adopted a lactose-free diet report that they don't lose a lot of pounds, but their weight naturally redistributes itself. They become more muscular and that unhealthy "spare tire" around their middles is reduced.

Personally, I lost twenty-five pounds without trying. Before adopting a lactose-free lifestyle, I was 210 pounds and working out consistently. I looked okay, but I wasn't losing as much weight as I would have expected, given how much exercise I was getting.

But on a lactose-free diet, I went down to 185 pounds. I feel like a million dollars. These days, I bet I eat twice as many calories a day as I used to. I eat a lot of fruit and a lot of bread. I love peanut butter and banana sandwiches. And I can't put a pound on.

What I've concluded is that diet contributes more to our overall health than exercise does. Exercising regularly is good for your muscles, bones, and mental state. But all the exercise in the world doesn't matter as much as your choices about how you fuel your body.

All that being said, I wouldn't want anyone to adopt a lactose-free diet simply to lose (or redistribute) body weight. This is not a weight-loss program. I ***do not recommend*** that you try lactose-free living for a few weeks or months, lose some pounds, and then go back to drinking milk and eating cheese and butter.

Why? Because if you do that, your lymphatic system will become clogged with lactose again. That means the system will no longer be functioning at its peak performance level. It will no longer be able to help your body use its fuel sources efficiently.

And the weight will pile right back on.

Do I Have To Do This 100%?

My not-so-simple answer to this is – I don't know. Remember, all of this is theory, based on my own experience and that of others. What I've observed – and learned in discussing this topic with other lactose-free individuals – is that removing any lactose from your diet will likely help you feel better. But I believe you need to follow a 100% lactose-free diet to see effects like I've experienced.

That being said, whether you go 100% or not, I believe that removing *any* significant amount of lactose from your diet will benefit you. My theory is that with less lactose in your system, your lymphatic traffic jam will shrink. It may not completely clear up the traffic jam, but the system will work more efficiently when it's not clogged with so much lactose.

Here's my advice: try going 100% lactose-free for two months. Then assess your results. Chances are, you'll feel so great and be so used to eating lactose-free, you won't want to back off.

The Bottom Line on Changing Your Diet

All of us know (or maybe we've been) people who tried various eating plans and cleanses that involve eliminating multiple food types all at once: gluten, sugar, dairy, and more. These plans often have great results in the short-term. People lose weight, have more energy, and feel healthier.

Advocates of these plans will give you a variety of reasons why they work, but I believe there's only one reason for their success: *because dairy is one of the foods you're required to stop eating.*

The problem is, most of these plans are difficult to maintain long-term. They simply ask us to give up too much of what we love. So we fall back into old habits, and before we know it, we're right where we were before we went on the plan or did the cleanse.

Lactose-free living is different. *I advocate a lactose-free diet as a lifelong change* – not as something to do only for a few weeks or months.

Why have I (and many others) been able to maintain a lactose-free diet over the long-term? The reasons are two-fold:

A lactose-free diet provides the same benefits as programs that require you to give up many other food types at the same time as you give up dairy.

Eating lactose-free over the long term is easier than a short-term elimination of multiple foods you love. Because you are only eliminating one thing – and because there are so many delicious, satisfying substitutes – it's much easier to maintain a permanently lactose-free diet.

What have you got to lose? Go ahead – give lactose-free living a try! I'm convinced you'll be delighted with the results.

Lactose-Free Stories: *Luke*

Luke is another brother of mine. (Remember, I have eight siblings; there's no shortage of stories about them!) Luke is fifty-six years old.

In late 2016, Luke had a heart attack. This was shortly before I discovered lactose-free living. But once I made my lifestyle change, I called Luke to talk about it. I shared my theory about the effects of lactose on the immune system with him and persuaded him to give it a try. When you're in a compromised position like Luke was, you're more apt to think – why not? What's there to lose?

Long story short: within a few months, Luke lost fifty-five pounds. Before beginning a lactose-free lifestyle, he'd suffered with continually watery eyes and a perpetual cough. Both of these conditions went away on Luke's 100% lactose-free diet.

This lasted into late 2017. Then, over the holidays, Luke had some dairy. That set him on a path back into the habit of eating dairy regularly. He wasn't going overboard, but he wasn't 100% anymore.

So what happened? Within six weeks, Luke's cough and watery eyes had returned. He gained back twenty-five of the fifty-five pounds he'd lost. Currently, he's working on getting back to being 100% lactose-free, but he's not quite there yet.

I share this story because – as I said above – I can't tell you what will happen to you personally if you give up some dairy but do not go 100% lactose-free. I can only tell you that in Luke's case, there was a huge difference between "some" and 100%.

Lactose-Free Stories: *Herbert*

I've already talked a bit about my dad, Herbert. He passed away less than a year ago. Not a day goes by that I don't miss him.

Honestly, we were lucky to have him as long as we did. He was eighty-five when he died, and he'd already survived three heart attacks. But toward the end, his health deteriorated rapidly. His heart was very weak. He could only walk halfway across a room before he ran out of breath. I took my son to visit shortly before my dad died, and seeing my dad's condition was a shock. His body was retaining excessive amounts of fluid and he was in a lot of pain. It was gut-wrenching to witness.

I don't think my dad had to die that way. His body shouldn't have had to work so hard, at the end. He shouldn't have suffered like that.

My dad was – and my mom still is – extremely religious. When I spoke with my dad near the end of his life, we talked about Jesus. At that point I'd been thinking a lot about Jesus – who He really was.

In Jesus's time, there was so much disease. If you were sick, people thought it was because you were a sinner. But Jesus was known as the Healer. He was the man who could heal the sick.

And how did Jesus heal people? He took them into the wilderness and fasted with them. The duration of a fast with Jesus was that famous length of time – the one every Christian knows because it's the amount of time from Ash Wednesday until Easter – forty days.

After John the Baptist baptized him, Jesus went alone into the desert and fasted for forty days. His fast wasn't what we usually think of when consider giving up something for Lent. Jesus didn't stop smoking or eating candy. He didn't go meatless and instead order the fish fry on Fridays.

Fasting, in Jesus's time, meant that for forty days, you gave up four things: oil, meat, wine – and dairy. If you took those four things out of your diet for forty days, Jesus said, you would be healed.

To me, this is all about the dairy. Jesus was onto something.

What my body went through when I stopped eating dairy was healing. Warts falling off, dandruff and eczema going away, congestion disappearing. That list of nineteen ailments I used to have but no longer do? That's healing.

That's not a pill. That is my body healing itself.

When I look back, it took about six weeks of lactose-free living – just over forty days – for me to notice enormous changes in my health.

This is precisely what Jesus would have predicted, two thousand years ago.

Toward the end of my dad's life, I talked about this with him. I asked, "What does fasting during Lent mean to you? Why do people do it?"

He said, "I guess it's to get healthy. You stay away from the bad stuff and you get healthy."

"That's exactly right," I said. "Do you know the origin of the word 'fast'?"

He shook his head.

"It means," I told him, "*to strengthen or make firm.*"

It was like a lightbulb went off in my dad's head. I just needed to explain it in terms he could understand. He could relate to it because of his Catholicism.

I only wish I could have convinced him sooner. He lived a good long life, but I wish he hadn't suffered so much at the end.

Lactose-Free Stories: *Ryan*

For an example of someone who has successfully stuck with a

lactose-free lifestyle, we need look no further than my friend Ryan. He's a thirty-six year old white man. He's been eating 100% lactose-free for over a year.

I asked him to send me a list of his health benefits, and this was his response:

- Healthy weight loss
- Improved digestive system
- Better functioning immune system
- Increased energy
- Increased focus
- "I just feel better"

Ryan loves to talk about this. He relishes telling people about his lactose-free lifestyle. And with the results he's had, I can certainly see why!

Chris's Lactose-Free Takeaways

You *can* eat lactose-free and enjoy a satisfying, healthy diet. Here's how:

- To learn what contains lactose and what's lactose-free, **read food labels, allergen menus, and ingredient lists on medications.**
- Understand that **plant-based products may taste different from their dairy-based counterparts** – but that doesn't mean they're not delicious.
- **Think of this as a permanent lifestyle change, not a short-term diet.**

CHAPTER 9

WHY THIS MATTERS TO ME: THE SALT RIVER PIMA-MARICOPA INDIAN COMMUNITY

What is the Salt River Pima-Maricopa Indian Community?
At this point I'd like to switch gears a bit. We've discussed how I became "accidentally lactose-free" and how I developed a theory about the effects of lactose on the immune system. I've provided tips to help you get started with a lactose-free lifestyle of your own. I've shared my own journey, as well as those of others who have adopted a lactose-free diet.

Now I want to talk about why I wrote this book in the first place. I wrote it for a group of people near and dear to me: the Salt River Pima-Maricopa Indian Community, or **SRPMIC**. To simplify matters, in this chapter I'm going to call them **the Community.**

The Community are a tribe in central and southern in Arizona. They're also called **Akimel O'otham,** which means "river people," because traditionally they lived near rivers. The casino I work for is on a Community reservation, and I have many friends and coworkers who are of Community descent.

When I began learning about the effects of lactose on the immune system, my primary goal was to help the Community people whom I work with.

Why? Because as a group, the modern-day Community's health is severely compromised:

- They have a diabetic rate of 34.2% (for men) and 40.8% (for women). This is compared to a 9.3% diabetic rate in the U.S. general population and a 16% diabetic rate in among all Native Americans tribes.
- Their obesity rates are 65 to 75% of the population.
- Their stomach cancer rate, compared to whites, is three times higher.

Now that you understand my theory about the effects of lactose on the immune system, I'll bet it comes as no surprise that ***I believe there's a strong correlation between the Community's diet and their health.***

History of the SRPMIC

Before the late 1600s, the Community had no interaction with non-Native people. Their way of life was based on their proximity to the river. They fished. They hunted game that also depended on the river to thrive. Their ancestors created complex systems of canals and ditches, using the precious river water to grow basic crops – corn, squash, and so on.

Even after outsiders arrived, the Community's contact with them was limited. For nearly the next two hundred years, the Community was left alone by most non-Natives, many of whom had no interest in the hot, arid region that makes up modern-day southern Arizona.

In 1853, the United States purchased southern Arizona from Mexico. At first this worked well for the Community, who traded with the many whites making their way toward the riches and plenty of California. But after the Civil War, many white Americans came to settle in the region where the Community lives.

Not long afterward, in the 1880s, the U.S. government put the Community on a reservation and dammed the river about fifty miles upstream of their reservation. The government did this to provide irrigation to others' land – some whites and some other Native tribes. But it dried up the Community land.

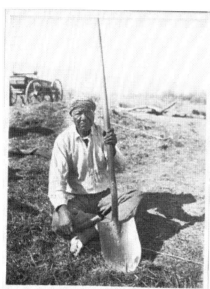

SRPMIC farmer, circa 1900

To this day, many in the Community call it a genocide. By removing their access to the river that was vital to their way of life, the government took away the Community's crop farming and fishing – their traditional food sources.

Without means to procure or grow their own food, the Community became reliant on government-supplied food – including dairy products. Before this, the Community had not consumed dairy as part of their diet.

And what was the effect? In a word – staggering. In photos from the 1880s to early 1900s, you can see Community people who don't exist anymore. They're strong and fit. But within a few generations, things changed dramatically. Today, most in the Community don't look anything like this.

Food and Health: My Connection with the Community

After figuring out my theory about the connection between lactose ingestion and the immune system, I was eager to show the Community how they would benefit from a lactose-free diet.

Sounds simple, right? But it isn't. As a white man, I can't just walk onto Native land and ask to speak to their board of directors. There's no access for me to anyone within the Community who is in a position of influence.

That's the reason I wrote this book. My hope is that with this information in book form, I can take it to the Community and ask them to consider what I have to say. My greatest wish is to help members of the Community make dietary changes leading to the health improvements that so many of them desperately need and desire.

Other Ethnicities

The Community is not the only group that struggles with health issues. But they're a perfect example of what happens when people exchange their native diet for a westernized, high-lactose diet.

Remember the lactase persistence map in Chapter 3? Go take another look. You'll notice something extraordinary: *most of the people who do NOT have lactase persistence – that is, those whose bodies no longer produce the enzyme lactase post-weaning – are natives of areas OTHER than Northern Europe.* And Northern Europeans, by heritage, are generally fair-skinned white people.

In other words, those without lactase persistence are primarily people of color.

What does this mean? It means that people of color – principally people of color in the western world who have adopted a typical western diet – are suffering health consequences in staggering numbers. This is true for many Native Americans, as well as for many other Americans who are people of color.

My focus and drive has been Native Americans – particularly the Community – because they're the people I work with every day. But this issue affects other ethnicities as well.

Please know that in no way do I blame anyone who must rely wholly or in part on cheap and/or government-sponsored food supplies for the state of their diet. The Community knew perfectly well how to eat healthfully – but through no fault of their own, their means to do so was destroyed. In one way or another, this is true for many groups.

Why? Because in the United States, much of our inexpensive and/or government-sponsored food supply is dairy-based.

For people with lactase persistence – i.e., many of Northern European descent – this might not be as much of a problem, regardless of their income level. But for people of color who also have limited incomes (and thus limited food choices), the problem is profound.

I don't presume to have a solution to this problem. But I *do* hope that by identifying the problem, I can work with others toward finding solutions.

Lactose-Free Stories: *Winter*

Winter is a Community member who is about thirty years old. He's one of the few people of Community descent (whom I know of) who follows a strict lactose-free diet.

So what does he look like? Well, photos don't lie. Here's a picture of Winter.

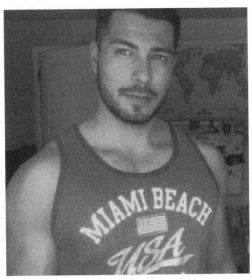

Winter Wood

What do you think?

I'd say Winter looks like what most of us think of when we conjure old-time images of Native Americans in our head. He looks like a picture of a Native male from a hundred and fifty years ago. We've all seen pictures like that – men who are sharp-featured and muscular, not an ounce of extra flesh anywhere on their bodies.

Members of the Community – members of all Native tribes – are 100% lactose-intolerant. Every single one of them has issues with lactose, whether those issues manifest as digestion troubles or not.

And yet, the vast majority of twenty-first century Native people eat dairy as a regular part of their diets.

Winter has discovered the benefits of a lactose-free diet and has tried to bring this message to other Community members. But it's difficult to reach them in large numbers. And it's difficult to help them change their diets when they have relied on government-provided food sources for such a long time.

Lactose-Free Stories: *Josephine*

At the casino, I work with a woman named Josephine who is of Community descent. She's twenty years old. Some time ago, I noticed that Josephine seemed to have lost quite a bit of weight. So I asked her about it.

"What have you been doing?" I said to her. "What have you done to lose so much weight?"

"For the past year," she replied. "I've eaten only fruits and vegetables."

I commend her for losing weight, but here's the thing: eating nothing but fruits and vegetables is an extreme way to do that. And I believe it's unnecessary. By eating this way, Josephine took a lot of nutrients out of her diet that her body needed – and she abstained from foods that would help her feel full and satisfied.

In my opinion, there was only one dietary change that made a difference: when Josephine ate only ate fruits and vegetables, obviously she wasn't ingesting lactose. That's why she lost weight. Good for her for doing it, but I believe she made it much harder on herself than it had to be.

A few months later, again I talked with Josephine about her diet. I asked, "How are things going? Are you feeling healthy?"

"Yes," she replied. "I feel great. I haven't been sick at all." She smiled at me and said, "But I *have* been cheating."

"Oh?" I said. "How are you cheating?"

"I've been eating bread lately."

"Is that bad?" I asked her. "Did bread do something bad to you before?"

"I have a gluten allergy," she told me. "I could never eat bread. It would give me a really bad reaction."

"But now you're eating it and you feel fine?"

"Yes," Josephine said. "I can eat bread and there's nothing happening. It's awesome."

"Interesting," I responded. "It sounds to me like your immune system is running perfectly these days. There's no more improper immune response to that allergen – to gluten."

I went on, "It's not that you can't have gluten. That was never the problem. The problem was, *when your immune system wasn't functioning properly, your body had a response to gluten.* But now that you're not eating lactose and your immune system is functioning at one hundred percent, your body is not responding negatively to gluten, the way it once did."

Chris's Lactose-Free Takeaways

The Salt River Pima-Maricopa Indian Community (SRPMIC, or the Community) are my friends and coworkers. Here's what I believe about their diet and health:

- **Traditionally, the Community ate healthfully – by fishing, hunting, and crop farming.**
- When the government took away their traditional means of acquiring food, instead providing them with government-sponsored food, **the Community began eating dairy – and ever since, their health has suffered tremendously.**
- **Other ethnic groups face the same issue.** People of color in the western world who have adopted a typical, dairy-heavy western diet are suffering health consequences in staggering numbers.

CHAPTER 10

WRAPPING IT UP IN A LACTOSE-FREE PACKAGE

Who am I to Give Nutritional Advice?

I know I've already said this, but it bears repeating: I'm not a doctor or a scientist. I can't offer you scientific evidence of the benefits to your immune system of eating a lactose-free diet. (But I *can* say that while the medical and scientific industries have not proven this, they haven't disproven it, either.)

What I have to offer you is my theory, based upon practices that not just me, but people from all walks of life, have put into place. Following a lactose-free diet has resulted in dramatic health improvements, both for myself and for the many others I've mentioned in this book.

Why not you, too?

Your Starting Point Doesn't Matter

This is what I believe.

Your current health status – whether you're fit or not, whether you struggle with health issues or not – doesn't matter at all. The decision to begin following a lactose-free diet doesn't have anything to do with an individual's health history.

Everyone can take this approach, because everyone will see a positive effect.

I can't tell you what your individual results will be. Each person is different, and each person's immune system responds differently to positive nutritional changes.

What I'm quite sure of – what I believe 100% -- is that if you give lactose-free living a try, you *will* see positive results.

Why We Don't Need Lactose

Just a recap:

- The *disaccharide lactose* is found every lactating female mammal's milk.
- Every young mammal produces the *enzyme lactase,* until the young mammal weans.
- Lactase enables mammals to break down lactose into the simple sugars *glucose* and *galactose.*
- For all mammals except humans, *production of lactase stops at weaning.*
- Some humans have developed *lactase persistence* – the ability to produce lactase post-weaning.
- *Lactase persistence varies greatly* from person to person. It is dependent on genetics, ethnicity, and age.
- Without lactase persistent, *our post-weaning bodies cannot break down lactose.*
- Gastrointestinal issues are common for people whose bodies no longer produce lactase – but *ingesting lactose without experiencing gastrointestinal issues does not guarantee that one's body still produces lactase.*
- In my opinion, *intact lactose has a profoundly detrimental effect on the lymphatic system (a key component of the immune system).*

Think about it: our dogs aren't sitting around drinking glasses of milk. They'd never do that (nor would they want to), because dogs, like all other mammals except humans, have never developed lactase persistence.

What's Wrong With Milk From an Animal?

Nothing – if you're that animal's offspring!

But what we have to keep in mind is, while the milk of all lactating female mammals contains lactose, ***an animal's milk is not the same as human milk.***

A lactating mother's milk is designed to feed that mother's young.

What does a newborn cow weigh? On average, a hundred pounds. Visualize that "baby." That hundred-pound newborn, with its thousand-pound mother, isn't the same as a seven-pound human newborn with a one-hundred-and-thirty-pound human mother.

When you drink cow's milk, you're drinking what a cow feeds her child. That "child" will grow several hundred pounds in its first few months of life. Why? Because nature designed a cow's milk to help a calf grow – perfectly, quickly, and exponentially.

Nature did *not* design that food source for us.

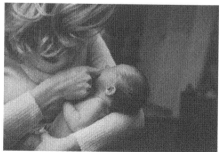

At this age, human mother's milk is the perfect food...

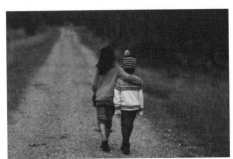

But by this age, there are many, much healthier options.

What Does the Lymphatic System Have to Do With It?

What happened to me is crystal clear. When I stopped ingesting dairy products, my lymphatic system (part of the immune system) changed. Every other change I experienced was part of a cascade effect – the result of my immune system functioning as it was intended to.

Ironically, when it comes to health, the immune system – the key to *all* health – is rarely discussed. There is endless talk about keeping our other systems functioning well – the circulatory system, the respiratory system, and so on. People are prescribed medications every day to address issues with these systems. Researchers work tirelessly to find ways to keep these systems performing capably.

But there is little discussion about what actually protects you, cleans you, and mends you.

I believe that when the lymphatic system is clogged with lactose, everything shuts down. A system that's supposed to be running like a racecar is running like a turtle. It's still running, but it's not doing so proficiently.

So what does lactose-free living do? It enables the lymphatic system to:

- Easily clear out cellular waste
- Efficiently repair damaged body parts (both those you can see and those you can't)
- Fiercely fight disease

One thing I want to be clear about: I do not believe that lactose in the lymphatic system causes cancer or causes one to get the flu. But I do believe that lactose in the lymphatic system prevents the body from fighting these and other issues effectively.

Where Do We Go From Here?

My advice is to give it a try! Take lactose completely out of your diet for two months. It might take some getting used to, but once you see the positive results, you won't want to go back to that occasional piece of cheese, glass of milk, or container of yogurt.

Those results, that wonderful feeling you'll have – the increased energy, focus, and overall good health, not to mention whatever positive changes you experience individually – will drive you to stay lactose-free.

Just give it a chance! Try 100% lactose-free living for two months – and after that, I'll bet you'll never touch that stuff again.

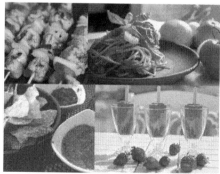

Just a few of the foods you can enjoy on a lactose-free diet.

Chris's Lactose-Free Takeaways

I'm not a doctor or scientist, but I believe I've discovered an explanation for the health issues that afflict so many people. Here's my theory:

- **Very few people maintain lactase persistence into adulthood.** The small intestines of most of the world's human population cannot break down lactose into glucose and galactose.
- **Lactose finds its way into the lymphatic system, clogging the system and preventing it from doing its jobs** of fighting large and small infections and diseases, as well as removing cellular waste.
- **The key to great health is to remove lactose from one's diet.** This allows the immune system (of which the lymphatic system plays a significant role) to do its job of maintaining complete health.

Stay in Touch!

I'd love to hear your lactose-free story. Please email me at lactosefreechris@gmail.com.

Thanks and happy lactose-free living!

REFERENCES

i. https://commons.wikimedia.org/wiki/File:Lactose_tolerance_in_the_Old_World.svg

ii. https://www.cancer.gov/about-cancer/causes-prevention/risk/age

iii. https://www.huffingtonpost.com/kathy-freston/vegan-diet-cancer_b_2250052.html

iv. https://www.cancer.gov/about-cancer/understanding/statistics

v.   https://commons.wikimedia.org/wiki/File:Lymph_nodes_illustration.jpg

vi. https://pets.webmd.co/dogs/guide/dogs-and-cancer-get-the-facts#1

vii. http:/www.washington.ed/new/2006/03/02/seeking-to-reduce-cancer-in-native-americans/

viii. https://commons.wikimedia.org/wiki/File:RECALLED_-_Cookies_(6322271441).jpg.

ix. https://www.niddk.nih.gov/health-information/health-statistics/overweight-obesity

x.   https://www.researchgate.net/publication/315772355_Policy_and_Social_Factors_Influencing_Diabetes_among_Pima_Indians_in_Arizona_USA

xi. http://commonsciencespace.com/gila-river-people/

xii. https://www.americanindiancancer.or/american-indian-cancer-facts

xiii. https://commons.wikimedia.org/wiki/File:Pima_Indian_man,_Miguel,_a_farmer,_Pima,_Arizona,_ca.1900_(CHS-3625).jpg

ACKNOWLEDGMENTS

Rachelle Reese
Without you, this would have never been. Thank you for saving
my life...I love you with all my heart...forever.

Dallas smith
Thank you for incessantly listening..these ideas may never have
come to light without you and the patio ;)

Young Chris Reese
Thank you for not thinking I'm crazy.

Mikkella Reese
Thank you for your beautiful brilliant young mind.

Quentin Krajnak
You are a son to me and I truly thank you for believing...all out of
the goodness of your heart.

Elizabeth Ede
Thank you for taking care of mom.

Nicholas Reese
Thank you for your ear and your insight brother...but especially
for being my brother.

Melissa Reese
Thank you for allowing me to borrow some of your tremendous courage...your heart amazes me.

Garrick Edison
Thank you for ALWAYS being you. You are the most talented respectful young man I have ever met. Believe.

Jade Hollis
Thank you for your gigantic talented heart..now we can go talk to your dad.

Hua Chen
Thank you for listening with an open mind and 'politely nudging' me in the right direction ;)

Dr. Snyder
Thank you for listening to my story..and for your unbelievable words of encouragement.

Colin Graham
Thank you for your imagination...It's beautiful.

Mark Graham
Thank you for taking the time to truly listen. I knew I was in the right place the first time I spoke with you.

Cynthia Swanson
Thank you for living this book with me and believing...words will never be enough to thank you. I am forever in your debt.

56411014R00071

Made in the USA
Columbia, SC
24 April 2019